BEYOND IMPLEMENTATION:

A Prescription for the Adoption of Healthcare Technology

Heather A. Haugen, PhD
Charles L. Fred

Todd Stansfield, Editor
Inbal C. Vuletich, Editor

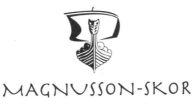

MAGNUSSON-SKOR
PUBLISHING, LLC

Denver
www.magnussonskor.com

Published by

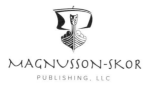

MAGNUSSON-SKOR
PUBLISHING, LLC

Magnusson-Skor Publishing
4600 S. Ulster Street Suite 1050
Denver, CO 80237
www.magnussonskor.com

Library of Congress Cataloging-in-Publication Data

Haugen, Heather A., 1973-
Fred, Charles L., 1961-
Ed. Todd Stansfield
Ed. Inbal Vuletich

    Beyond Implementation: A Prescription for the Adoption of Healthcare Technology.
    p. cm.
    Includes biographical references.
    ISBN 978-0-9842051-4-1
    1. Healthcare Technology Adoption 2. EHR adoption 3. Healthcare
    4. Health Information Technology I. Title

Second Edition

This book is dedicated to our colleagues
at The Breakaway Group

CONTENTS

P R E F A C E

Our journey to understand the factors that drive successful electronic health record (EHR) adoption began in 2009 when the Health Information Technology for Economic and Clinical Health (HITECH) Act led to a historic increase in implementations. At that time only 12 percent of non-federal acute care hospitals and only 48 percent of provider practices had installed an EHR system (Office for the National Coordinator on Health Information Technology, 2015). In the span of seven years, those numbers have climbed dramatically, with over 96 percent of non-federal acute care hospitals using a certified EHR and 83 percent of provider practices using an EHR application. Today the challenge is not implementing clinical information systems, but adopting those that have already been installed. Healthcare organizations now face the continuous challenge of helping their employees use these applications to provide patient care despite system upgrades, employee turnover, workflow enhancements, competing priorities, and resource shortages.

The second edition of *Beyond Implementation* examines the primary reasons for poor and failed EHR adoption, explores the outcomes of healthcare organizations, and reveals a new approach for successful adoption and lasting value. The original research published in the first edition remains relevant to the challenges in healthcare; however, since the book's development we have learned more about the challenges and strategies of replacing an existing EHR – a trend we explore and address in our analysis. At the time of the first book our industry was primarily transitioning from paper to clinical information systems. Now organizations are increasingly looking to replace legacy and disparate applications with today's enterprise systems.

One example is Medical Center Health System (MCHS) headquartered in Odessa, Texas. MCHS sought to replace its legacy EHR application with a new system across both the ambulatory and acute care settings. MCHS serves as a timely example of the focus and effort required to replace a legacy EHR system with a robust enterprise clinical information system. A year before the go-live event the organization began planning for adoption with joint leadership and ownership of the strategic initiative between IT and clinical leadership. MCHS committed to engage and support end users in the process, provide relevant and valuable education, track and measure performance, and sustain these efforts into the future.

Through our research and extensive experience with healthcare organizations, this book investigates the factors that drive improved clinical and financial outcomes from healthcare technology. Our key premise: a myopic focus on the implementation project impedes the adoption and long-term sustainment of an EHR application.

The State of the Industry
"In the last seven years, our industry has evolved significantly to embrace new advancements in technology . . . The story is richer and more complex . . . and this complexity derives from the trial and

error of helping over 1 million clinicians – roughly a third of U.S. providers – adopt clinical information systems . . . We want to help healthcare organizations shift from the discontinuous and episodic actions of an implementation to the ongoing process and discipline of adoption. The good news is that we are smarter now and more aware of both the challenges and the opportunities that exist for the systemic use of an electronic health record."

Implementation vs. Adoption

"Implementation happens when the application is installed and live; an important milestone from a technology perspective, but only a small step toward adoption. Adoption is the continuous process of keeping users informed and engaged, providing innovative ways for them to become proficient in new tasks quickly, measuring changes in critical outcomes, and striving to sustain that level of performance long-term. Adoption is not a snapshot at a single point in time; it is a motion picture."

The Potential of EHR

"Today, we now find ourselves beyond the tipping point as leaders, healthcare professionals, and patients are completely invested in their EHR and the data they contain. Again, our industry faces another critical turning point where simply implementing a clinical information system is not enough. Organizations now must look to improve outcomes using technology."

Preventing "Go-Live Myopia"

"When decision-makers focus on just one event, a successful go-live, it is very easy to forego the processes that ensure adoption. Too many organizational leaders still believe that once the application goes live, users will embrace it. However, it becomes strikingly obvious after a go-live when the key elements of adoption have been left out. Many organizations have implemented an EHR, but very few have successfully adopted the EHR."

How Leaders Create a "Tone at the Top"

"Leaders currently in charge of EHR adoption need to develop a ferocious understanding of what they are going to stop doing, and then maintain the courage to follow through on their decisions. Because it demonstrates active commitment to end users who are affected by the new workflows, this may be the single greatest action toward successful adoption of an EHR."

A Simulation-Based Approach

". . . simulators literally change how healthcare providers learn new technology. First, they are designed separately for each role that will use the application . . . Individuals do not have to learn to use every function of the application – the focus of traditional vendor training – but they do have to learn all functions related to their specific role. It is a mistake to teach every function of the entire application . . ."

Performance Metrics and Adoption

"The commitment to identify even just a few key metrics will provide enormous value to the organization. First, it will be very handy in proving meaningful use. Second, it can be used as a dashboard for measuring performance of the EHR for the life of the application. Most importantly it will drive continual improvement in the specific areas of value to the organization."

Planning for Sustainment

"Effective sustainability plans require resources, time and money. Keep in mind that adoption is never static . . . Leadership must plan for the investment and fund it if their ultimate goal is improved performance. Most organizations only achieve modest adoption after a go-live event, and it takes relentless focus to achieve the levels of adoption needed to improve quality of care, patient safety and financial outcomes."

A C K N O W L E D G E M E N T S

Developing this second edition has marked the next chapter in a rewarding and challenging adventure. Since first writing *Beyond Implementation* seven years ago, we are humbled by and thankful for the unwavering support we have received from healthcare professionals across the country, many of whom have confirmed the hardships of technology adoption and the value of the methodology that was borne out of the research. As our industry has evolved and experienced significant progress and more change, we recognized the need to update and refresh the original book. This new edition explores the current state of today's healthcare organizations and examines the industry's greatest challenges and opportunities to improve clinical and financial outcomes through technology.

Many colleagues and mentors have been vital to the creation of the first and second editions of *Beyond Implementation*. We would like to acknowledge the valuable work of Dr. Jeffrey R. Woodside, who served as a co-author of the first edition. Many of Dr. Woodside's significant contributions to the first edition remain relevant and have helped shape the direction of this second edition. Inbal Vuletich was also instrumental to the writing and editing of the first and second edition. Steven Burkett, former CEO of UT Medical Group, also contributed significantly to the development of the first edition by graciously sharing his organization's efforts around adoption. As the editor of the second edition, Todd Stansfield has served as the primary driver of this latest release of *Beyond Implementation*.

We would also like to thank and acknowledge the leadership team at HealthSouth for allowing us to share their incredible journey of adoption. In particular, we would like to express our gratitude to Mark Tarr, Executive Vice President and COO; Rusty Yeager, Senior Vice President and CIO; Tracy Foy, Vice President and CTO; Dayle Unger, Vice President of Clinical Transformation; Eileen Thayer, Clinical Liaison for Physicians, Case Management and Admissions; and Ellen Dandridge, Associate Director of CIS at HealthSouth.

The work being done by the leadership team at Medical Center Health System (MCHS) by William Webster, Chief Executive Officer, Gary Barnes, Chief Information Officer, and Dr. Arun Mathews, Chief Medical Information Officer, represents an important shift in paradigms for healthcare IT. The team has been instrumental in redefining how adoption of technology begins with leadership and planning prior to implementation.

Our acknowledgements would not be complete without recognizing the continued support of our family members who encourage us in our sometimes zealous commitment to making a difference in healthcare for clinicians and patients.

BEYOND IMPLEMENTATION:

A Prescription for the Adoption
of Healthcare Technology

INTRODUCTION

After finally passing through the security checkpoint in the Milwaukee International Airport (MKE), a frazzled traveler is greeted by a low-hanging placard. It reads: *Recombobulation Area.* Clearly someone on the MKE management team, someone with a sense of humor, acknowledged the fact that many travelers become a bit discombobulated attempting to make it through security and that an "area" is needed to get one's collective psyche back in order. No doubt similar thinking went into the airport code being MKE and not MIA. We've witnessed this sign many times during our travels, but today the message seems especially appropriate. The return trip followed a healthcare conference on Lake Geneva where a wide spectrum of thought leaders presented and discussed learnings from the past decade. A shared conclusion among the group is that no one could have prepared for or predicted the level of changes thrown at the healthcare environment over these past years. Now the worry is centered on what is coming next.

> "A shared conclusion among the group is that no one could have prepared for or predicted the level of changes thrown at the healthcare environment over these past years."

During a break at the conference an attendee approached us holding the first edition of *Beyond Implementation*. The sight was confirmation that healthcare leaders are still finding value in the research, amazing considering seven years had passed since its

2

publication. "Wonderful book," the woman said. "I just wish I'd known about it a few years ago when we were implementing our EHR. It would've saved us from many headaches and sleepless nights. Now we've got new challenges such as replacing our old system." She paused and glanced at the book. "You haven't written another one by any chance?"

Her comments provoked an uncomfortable realization: Our book, which lasted a considerable time on the Amazon Best Seller's List for Hospital Administration & Care, was now outdated. The Health Information Technology for Economic and Clinical Health (HITECH) Act, the Meaningful Use Incentive Program, the switch from paper to electronic – all no longer represent the world we are working in today. We recognized the need to update the book to reflect the significant progress made over the past few years, even though our original research and core method for adopting technology remain as relevant today as ever.

In the last seven years, our industry has evolved significantly to embrace new advancements in technology. Nearly a decade's worth of this story remains untold, which is the reason for this second edition. The story is richer and more complex than our first edition, and this complexity derives from the trial and error of helping over 1 million clinicians – roughly a third of U.S. providers – adopt clinical information systems. It also comes from the real-life examples of healthcare organizations leading this work.

> "The story is richer and more complex than our first edition..."

Among them is HealthSouth, one the largest providers of post-acute healthcare services in the country, which has undergone 98 implementations to date. No story would be complete without an examination of HealthSouth's innovative and relentless focus on key drivers of adoption such as leadership engagement.

Our fundamental goal remains the same as in our first edition: We want to help healthcare organizations shift from the discontinuous and episodic actions of an implementation to the ongoing process and discipline of adoption. The good news is that we are smarter now and more aware of both the challenges and the opportunities that exist for the systemic use of an electronic health record. It is time, however, for those of us that have lived through the tumult of the past decade to have a recombobulation area. We hope that this new edition of *Beyond Implementation* provides you that space.

"Much like luggage undergoing TSA screening at airports, providers have been subjected to intense scrutiny. While travelers submit to luggage x-rays, 3-ounce liquid restrictions, laptop scrutiny, shoeless pat-downs, similarly providers submit to coding reviews, software certifications, quality metrics, productivity measures, and patient-satisfaction ratings. A recombobulation area would be a welcome relief."

Dr. CT Lin, CMIO, University of Colorado Health

A Journey of Healthcare Technology Adoption

Chapter Preview:
- The HealthSouth Story
- Research Conclusions

6

The HealthSouth Story

HealthSouth, one of the nation's largest providers of inpatient rehabilitation services in the United States, faced a significant decision in 2009. The company was receiving (and continues to receive) approximately 90 percent of its patients from acute care hospitals, most of which were transitioning from paper to electronic health record (EHR) systems to pursue the government incentives offered through the Health Information Technology for Economic and Clinical Health (HITECH) Act. Though HealthSouth was not eligible for the incentives as a post-acute care company, it immediately recognized the value of investing in healthcare IT to support its acute-care partnerships and the coordination of care. Having the financial capacity to implement a new system across 98 inpatient rehabilitation hospitals, and recognizing the recent advancements in healthcare technology, HealthSouth embarked on a quest toward adopting its first-ever clinical information system. The move would prepare the organization for a rapidly evolving industry that was placing more emphasis on value-based, rather than fee-for-service-based, care. It would also provide the company with a platform to quickly respond to changes in government reimbursements, which generated most of its revenue. The journey to implement a clinical information system would begin by partnering with one of the few IT vendors with experience, investments, and interest in developing a customized EHR system for inpatient rehabilitation, Cerner. HealthSouth would purchase and brand the system "ACE IT" – Advancing Clinical Excellence through Information Technology – to encompass its vision and purpose.

Despite the resounding commitment from HealthSouth's leadership, the overall effort would prove to be one of the most challenging in recent years. At this time, the company operated 98 inpatient rehabilitation hospitals, each with minor but still important variations in workflow and processes. Because all hospitals would undergo an implementation, HealthSouth needed to develop a scalable, repeatable implementation model that would not only be effective and efficient, but would keep costs within the organization's operating and capital budgets. The sheer size and scope of the overall effort would necessitate staggered implementations over the course of several years and a relentless commitment to a long-term approach. Additionally, HealthSouth was expanding and actively building new, or de novo, hospitals, which would also be included in the project. Unlike existing facilities, de novo hospitals often employ acute care professionals with no experience in rehabilitation therapy or working for HealthSouth. These professionals would need additional education and support beyond the transition from paper to electronic health records.

In 2010 HealthSouth began the first of three pilot implementations at a de novo hospital. The first pilot would serve as an early and important lesson in the significant work that lay ahead.

HealthSouth sought to uncover the most important aspects of implementing ACE IT and develop an effective, accurate and standardized approach for supporting other hospitals going forward. Recognizing the importance of education, HealthSouth also sought to define and solidify its training model.

The first pilot hospital demonstrated the considerable learning challenges of a de novo hospital. HealthSouth needed to provide significant onsite support to prepare users, many of whom were grappling with learning the new system as well as orienting to rehabilitation workflows and documentation processes. The extent of this early effort illustrated the challenge of implementing the system at scale. As planned, HealthSouth spent the remainder of the year developing a scalable, repeatable model to rollout the system effectively across the organization, as well as evaluating the system and the details of a long-term contract with Cerner.

When the summer of 2011 arrived, HealthSouth was ready for its second pilot implementation. This time the effort would occur at an existing inpatient hospital converting from paper to the EHR system. Unlike the first hospital, the leadership team and staff had significant rehabilitation experience and thus only needed to transition from paper to electronic processes. The hospital also demonstrated quality communication practices and engagement from employees. Additionally, HealthSouth had developed a 10-week implementation cycle to accommodate a mass rollout of ACE IT. The company sought to test the new model that among other things relied on super-user coaches and classroom education.

Although the second implementation required less onsite

support than the first, the company discovered challenges with its classroom education model. While ultimately demonstrating quality outcomes, super-user training illustrated the difficulty of accommodating different learning styles in a classroom setting. The variation in learning styles, needs, and retention was greater for the general end-user population, some of whom continued to focus on basic navigation while others learned more advanced tasks. The variation in knowledge and confidence in the system carried over to the go-live event and demonstrated the need for a more uniform, targeted, and effective approach to education.

The 10-week implementation cycle would be put to its greatest test in October of that same year, when HealthSouth implemented ACE IT at a second de novo hospital. A pattern similar to the first de-novo implementation emerged: Users struggled not only to learn the EHR within the context of their role, but the workflow, responsibilities, and nuances of rehabilitation therapy. Teaching and learning styles varied significantly in the classroom which made it difficult to adhere to the 10-week implementation cycle. Communication and raising awareness around the project were also challenges. Another challenge was overcoming the myopic focus on the go-live event, which distracted from the need to and importance of sustaining the effort beyond the implementation.

Yet by 2012 HealthSouth's leadership team remained relentless in its vision to implement ACE IT. The organization sought a new approach to realize lasting value from the application. This time the new approach would shift the focus from merely implementing ACE IT to the critical factors that drive healthcare technology adoption; mainly, leadership engagement, targeted education, performance metrics, and sustainment of the overall effort. Implementation happens when the application is installed and live; an important milestone from a technology perspective, but only a small step toward adoption. Adoption is the continuous process of keeping users informed and engaged, providing innovative ways for them to become proficient in new tasks quickly, measuring changes in critical outcomes, and striving to sustain that level of performance long-term. Adoption is not a snapshot at a single point in time; it is a motion picture. The new approach would lead to 98 successful implementations to date, a remarkable and staggering number expected to climb to 127 by 2018. So what has been HealthSouth's formula?

HealthSouth has remained relentlessly committed to the factors that drive EHR adoption. It has also developed strategies and an approach that is uniquely effective for its organization.

Central to HealthSouth's success has been its focus on developing and engaging leadership in the overall effort. At the national and regional levels, HealthSouth has engaged a physician advisory board, case management/quality board, and clinical leadership boards across nursing, pharmacy, and therapy to ensure use of the system produces optimal clinical outcomes. The health system's National Director of Nursing, National Director of Therapy Operations, National Director of Pharmacy Operations, HIMS directors, Case Management/Quality Director, and regional Business Office directors are also actively involved, and regularly communicate and participate in monthly change control calls. HealthSouth also holds weekly change control calls with its Senior Administrative team, which includes the Chief Nursing Officer (CNO), Director of National Therapy (DTO), Director of Pharmacy (DOP), HIMS Director, Vice President of Clinical Transformation, Vice President of IT and Associate Director of CIS. At the hospital level, the company has developed a standard process for engaging leadership. Each year HealthSouth holds a CEO Forum in December to educate and prepare hospital CEOs that are approaching an implementation the following year. Each CEO is required to review important adoption practices to generate awareness and start a dialogue with clinicians, as well as to learn from the challenges and successes of organizations who have previously engaged in this work. As an extension of hospital leadership, HealthSouth also develops coaches to provide at-the-elbow support to users before, during, and after go-live. Organizationally, HealthSouth has raised awareness and engagement through branding and ongoing communication, and continues to adhere to effective oversight and governance processes.

The company has also transformed how it educates users. Rather than restricting education to the classroom, HealthSouth relies primarily on simulation-based education that provides users with hands-on experience completing critical workflow tasks in a simulated EHR. This has ensured a consistent, relevant, repeatable, and accessible education experience and led to high levels of knowledge and confidence in the system. HealthSouth has also shortened classroom training and repurposed it to focus on supplemental topics and activities such as workflow considerations, policies and procedures. The result is users who are prepared to perform their role proficiently during and after go-live with minimal disruption.

Central to leadership's ability to govern and oversee the initiative has been HealthSouth's commitment to collecting performance metrics. The organization requires all users to complete 100 percent of their simulated-based education before attending classroom training and gaining access to the application. These metrics are available to leadership through an enterprise application that HealthSouth has branded "ACE IT Community." Additionally, the organization regularly collects performance metrics through its EHR system including data around computerized provider order entry (CPOE). The ACE IT Community not only provides leadership and users with performance data, but also 24/7 online access for users to simulation-based education, reference materials, and regular communication from leadership.

To ensure each hospital continues to use the application proficiently after go-live, HealthSouth has also committed to sustaining its efforts around leadership engagement, education, and performance metrics. Leadership continues to regularly communicate, oversee, and govern EHR use. HealthSouth continues to support its network of super-user coaches to ensure they can continue to effectively support users long after the go-live event. Additionally, access to education is ongoing for existing employees and a critical focus for onboarding new hires. Performance metrics continue to be captured, monitored, and used to make improvements.

HealthSouth has developed an implementation model that is

scalable and repeatable. Each implementation is managed and led by a seven-person interdisciplinary team including a coordinator, two nursing specialists, a physician specialist, a therapy specialist, a pharmacy specialist, and a generalist. Notably, this team provides clinical representation to lead the effort with involvement from IT. Each member provides support to a respective population of users, with the generalist focused on marketing, admissions, case management, and support of other departments. Because the company implements ACE IT across five hospitals at a time, HealthSouth has multiple teams to manage and support the go-live effort.

The members of the team facilitate the 10-week implementation cycle. The cycle is comprised of two-week segments devoted to one or more areas of focus. Before the start of the implementation cycle, each hospital receives a survey to capture important information such as overall hospital structure, number of employees and providers, and elected coaches. The coordinator of the implementation team also begins holding information calls with hospital leadership to answer questions and discuss the schedule and process for the implementation.

Once the 10-week implementation cycle begins, the focus shifts to capturing the current state workflows of the hospital, supplying the workflow data to the IT vendor, building the application, educating coaches, testing the application, and educating users before the go-live event. By documenting the current state workflows, the implementation team identifies any gaps that occur after converting from paper to an EHR system. By educating coaches weeks before users, the coaches are able to have adequate time to practice in the application training environment. The timing of end-user education is also designed to provide ample time for learners to practice in the training environment and prepare. By the time of the go-live event, hospital leadership, coaches, and users are prepared and proficient in the application.

Implementation Week	Description
Week One	• Document the current workflows and processes to identify important considerations for the application build • Identify potential gaps in processes that would occur after converting from paper to an EHR • Provide coach workshops • Provide simulation-based education to coaches"
Week Two	• Continue the onsite workflow assessment and also begin translating this information into the IT vendor's data collection workflows to build the system • Continue providing simulation-based education to coaches
Week Three	• Build the application • Provide education to coaches • Provide simulation-based education to users to complete 100 percent of assigned learning prior to scheduled classroom review sessions in Week 6 or Week 7

Implementation Week	Description
Week Four	• Build the application • Continue providing simulation-based education to users • Allow coaches to practice in the training environment
Week Five	• Test the application • Continue providing simulation-based education to users • Allow coaches to practice in the training environment
Week Six	• Test the application • Continue providing simulation-based education to users • Allow users to attend classroom review sessions once simulation-based education is complete • Allow coaches to practice in the system • Allow users to practice in the training environment after completing classroom review sessions
Week Seven	• Continue providing simulation-based education to users • Allow users to attend classroom review sessions once simulation-based education is complete • Coaches must attend at least one review session • Allow coaches to practice in the training environment • Allow users to practice in the training environment after completing classroom review sessions

Implementation Week	Description
Week Eight	• Continue providing simulation-based education to users • Allow users to attend classroom review sessions once simulation-based education is complete • Allow coaches to practice in the system • Allow users to practice in the training environment after completing classroom review sessions
Week Nine	• Go-Live
Week Ten	• Go-Live

Despite its achievements, the challenges and work to sustain EHR adoption are ongoing at HealthSouth. Leadership and employee turnover, application upgrades and workflow enhancements all threaten to erode HealthSouth's level of adoption. HealthSouth has experienced high levels of adoption only to see those levels fluctuate through natural changes to the organization and its clinical information system. Through its relentless commitment to adoption, however, HealthSouth has consistently demonstrated high levels of adoption.

HealthSouth stands as a pioneer and example to healthcare organizations engaged in this work. Much can be learned from analyzing the case study of this company. HealthSouth's relentless commitment to adopting ACE IT has prepared the organization to succeed in a healthcare industry seeking to improve clinical and financial outcomes. The publicly-traded company is now capable of responding to ever-evolving payment models and has prepared to engage in other innovative healthcare IT initiatives. Partnering with Cerner, HealthSouth has analyzed large data sets of its patient population and is now using predictive analytics to identify the leading causes of acute-care transfers to prevent them from occurring. HealthSouth is also focusing on other initiatives around managing population health.

Notably, HealthSouth's story illustrates not only the strategies that are uniquely successful to its organization, but the four main factors that drive adoption of all clinical information systems—leadership engagement, targeted education, performance metrics, and sustainment. The company attributes its success to its ongoing commitment to leadership, education and support of its coach network. This book explores these and other factors in depth through the lens and real-life examples of HealthSouth and other organizations. The result is a roadmap for every healthcare leader and professional engaged in this important work and striving to gain the most value from their clinical information systems.

Research Conclusions

1. Implementation and adoption are not synonymous, but almost universally treated as the same effort.
2. Very few organizations track end-user adoption in terms of clinical and financial outcomes.
3. Adoption is highly dependent on the degree of engaged leadership. Clinical leaders need to be involved early in the process and be empowered to make decisions that impact the use of the application.
4. Traditional training methods, like classroom training, don't produce proficient users. Inadequate education of users is a significant contributor to poor EHR adoption and ultimately poor business outcomes.
5. Successful organizations develop ongoing plans for sustaining adoption long past the implementation.

19

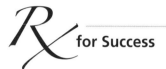**for Success**

- Put a strategy in play for adoption not just implementation.
- Learn from other healthcare organizations going through an EHR adoption. Visit other organizations that have been successful in their journey!
- Utilize research findings to overcome common barriers to EHR adoption.

The Imperatives for EHR Adoption

Chapter Preview:
- The economic and political pressures on healthcare are extraordinary.
- EHRs are a critical component of healthcare infrastructure.
- Adopting an EHR will improve the organization's quality of care, patient safety and efficiency.
- Adopting an EHR early gives the organization a competitive advantage.

There are risks and costs to a program of action, but they are far less than the long-range risks and costs of comfortable inaction."

~ John F. Kennedy

The most durable tools are created through the process of forging rather than casting. Using extreme heat and compression, metal is subjected to tremendous stress as it is shaped. Ironically, this tremendous stress is what actually creates the strength in the tool. Casting, on the other hand, is a fairly stress-free process in which the metal is simply poured into a mold and left to harden. As a result, it is brittle, and therefore not as strong or resilient as a forged metal product. Consider the application of this metaphor to the state of healthcare today. Through tremendous economic, political and consumer-driven stress, healthcare is literally being forged into a stronger and more resilient shape.

We continue to experience rising healthcare costs in the United States, which have climbed for over 50 years at an alarming rate. Between 1960 and 2013, total healthcare expenditures as a percentage of gross domestic product (GDP)

23

> **"Through tremendous economic, political and consumer-driven stress, healthcare is literally being forged into a stronger and more resilient shape."**

have more than tripled, from 5 to 17.4 percent, and they show no signs of slowing (Catlin & Cowan, 2015).

Figure 2.1: Total Expenditures on Health as a Percentage of GDP in the United States

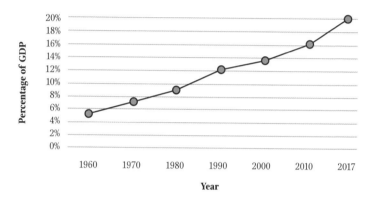

Today, we spend approximately 17.5 percent of our GDP on healthcare, making it the largest single sector of the economy, and this number is projected to surpass 20 percent by 2025 (Centers for Medicare & Medicaid Services, 2014). To fight rising healthcare costs, an abundance of new legislation has passed, continuing to create challenges for providers and other healthcare professionals. The Health Information Technology for Economic and Clinical Health (HITECH) Act, Physician Quality Reporting System (PQRS), and Medicare Access and Chip Reauthorization Act (MACRA) are all forcing providers to adapt to new rules, regulations and payment models to improve patient care (Medical Economics, 2015). Providers now face the most significant changes to provider reimbursement under Medicare since 1965

(Wolinsky, 2016). Meanwhile, providers continue to work long hours, averaging 51 each week in 2013 for all medically-related activities (Glicksman, 2013). These forces are changing the shape of healthcare by creating economic, political and social pressures on our industry. It is up to us to ensure the result is a stronger, more resilient healthcare system.

Since the passage of the American Recovery and Reinvestment Act (ARRA) of 2009, legislative changes have focused on using technology to improve the cost and effectiveness of healthcare. The ARRA allocated $59 billion to improving areas such as health IT, primary care provider training, chronic disease research, community health centers and research, and just over $19 billion in net appropriations for the HITECH Act. The ARRA and HITECH Act have laid the foundation for the wide-scale acquisition and use of EHR systems. Today at least 90 percent of hospitals across 44 states have attested to Meaningful Use criteria established through the HITECH Act for Medicare and Medicaid (Office of the National Coordinator for Health Information Technology, 2015). Additionally, two-thirds of Medicare-eligible providers attested to Meaningful Use Stage 1 as of 2013 (Office of the National Coordinator for Health Information Technology, 2014). Current and future legislation will continue to build on this progress and focus on improving quality of care and lowering costs through technology. In most cases, however, the legislation falls short of the vision, and the value comes from the work done at the local level in healthcare organizations. This emphasizes the need for organizations to adopt EHR systems.

EHRs are a critical component
of healthcare infrastructure

Both universal adoption of EHRs and interoperability are required to forge a more efficient and effective healthcare system. The Office of the National Coordinator (ONC) for Health Information Technology is tasked with creating a nationwide interoperable health information network to provide a secure infrastructure that connects healthcare providers and consumers (Nationwide Health Information Network, 2009). This is a mammoth undertaking, requiring oversight of everything from privacy and security to establishment of standards and certification processes, but it is a worthy cause in light of the potential benefits. The challenges the ONC faces are evident, considering that the position of national coordinator overseeing the ONC has been held by six different individuals since first being created in 2004 (Bazzoli, 2016).

A secure, interoperable health record, available to a patient anywhere in the country, depends on every clinician adopting an EHR. How might this vision directly benefit the organization?

- Imagine never treating a patient again without full knowledge of allergies, medications and previous medical history
- Imagine managing the care of chronically-ill patients with automatic screening reminders and evidence-based medicine guidelines
- Imagine having a complete health record available when covering for another provider's patients

26

- Imagine the ease of participating in insurers' pay-for-performance programs and other quality initiatives
- Imagine the decrease in medication errors and the time savings for providers who can electronically prescribe

EHR systems have already begun transforming healthcare by providing clinicians access to comprehensive health information that is secure, standardized and shared. Specifically, they promote increased healthcare quality, error prevention, reduced healthcare costs and increased efficiency.

> "EHR systems have already begun transforming healthcare by providing clinicians access to comprehensive health information that is secure, standardized and shared."

27

Adopting an EHR will improve the organization's quality of care, patient safety and efficiency

We have the opportunity to transform healthcare by providing clinicians and consumers with access to comprehensive health information that is secure, standardized and shared. A significant body of research confirms the value of EHRs in improving patient safety, improving coordination of care, enhancing documentation, reducing administrative inefficiencies, facilitating clinical decision-making and adherence to evidence-based guidelines (Chen et al., 2009). We will not spend time on a comprehensive literature review here, but we have included a summary of some of the most compelling literature in Appendix A that illustrates the evidence for improved outcomes.

A healthy dose of skepticism will serve us well as we review the EHR literature, not because it is misleading, but because it doesn't tell the whole story. Despite the promises of an EHR system, why do we continue to hear stories of end-user resistance, applications with configuration issues, workflow struggles, higher costs and lower revenues, increases in staffing and worse quality metrics? The disconnect between the evidence in the literature and our real-world experiences is borne in the assumption that implementing an EHR and adopting an EHR are synonymous.

The differences between implementing and adopting an EHR are evident when one examines data from the College of Health Information Management Executives (CHIME). Figure 2.2 shows the gap between implementation and adoption across several key functions of clinical information systems (Haugen, CHIME Focus Group, 2012). As you can see, the rate of adoption is significantly lower than the rate of implementation, illustrating that installing an EHR doesn't lead to adopting the application for the clinical benefit of users. The more complex functions, such as Computerized Provider Order Entry (CPOE) and Clinical Decision Support (CDS), have the biggest gap in adoption because they require the most significant changes in workflow.

Figure 2.2: Gaps between EHR Implementation and Adoption Across Key Functions

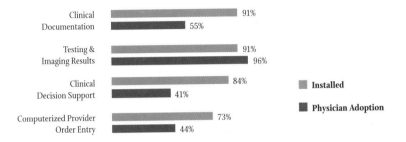

Adopting an EHR early gives the organization a competitive advantage

At the time of writing the first edition of *Beyond Implementation*, our industry faced a critical turning point in health information technology (HIT). The HITECH Act was causing a historic rise in EHR implementations across the country. Despite the growing demand for technology, we made the argument that the industry had yet to reach the "tipping point" in terms of accepting technology's role in healthcare – Gladwell's definition of that magic moment when an idea, trend, or social behavior crosses a threshold, tips, and spreads like wildfire (Gladwell, 2002). Now, we find ourselves beyond the tipping point as leaders, healthcare professionals, and patients are completely invested in their EHR and the data they contain. Again, our industry faces another critical turning point where simply implementing a clinical information system is not enough. Organizations must now look to improve outcomes using technology. As we examine in this second edition, adoption of these systems is the antecedent of improving clinical and financial outcomes, and for those willing to seize the opportunity, now is the time to break away.

Let's consider another metaphor. The mile run is a grueling track and field race that can easily be used as a metaphor to articulate a "breakaway"—an advantage created by purposely sprinting away from the group at a point when all runners are experiencing the greatest pain. Halfway through the notorious four-lap race, at the beginning of the third lap, the breakaway occurs. Up to this point, nearly all runners are still tightly packed together, jockeying for position, cruising at a pace that pushes each runner's pulse to between 160 and 190 beats per minute. Lactic acid is accumulating in the large leg muscles, lungs burn as they are filled to capacity and emptied every second, and each runner's brain constantly takes stock of the body's condition even as it craves oxygen for itself. At this point, every runner in the pack must make a very tough decision: to summon a burst of speed and attempt to win by breaking away from the other runners, or to let others go ahead and rationalize that winning is not really so important.

The breakaway is more than a physical action; it is the most significant mental challenge a runner faces. The runner must put all bodily pain and mental anguish aside if they are to break away and win. The breakaway lasts only 20 to 30 seconds, but it is devastating for those who choose to avoid it, and inspiring for those who choose to go faster and become part of the lead

30

pack. The leaders move continuously ahead of those left behind, drawing strength from the exhilarating sensation of actually being in a position to win. Their attention is focused outward, toward the future, on reaching the finish line first. Those who follow are immediately consumed by physical exhaustion and the deep disappointment of watching all opportunity for victory vanish. Their attention is focused inward, toward the past, on wondering why they didn't have the strength to stay with the leaders.

A similar phenomenon will occur in healthcare as many organizations compete in a relatively equal position of market share and growth, with comparable equipment and technological sophistication. Suddenly, one organization chooses to make a significant move to change the way they practice by rapidly adopting an EHR, leaving their competitors behind. Just like the runner who initiates the breakaway, a healthcare organization that quickly sets itself apart from its competitors becomes outwardly focused on winning. People in these organizations, especially clinicians, are typically more patient-centered, have higher morale and understand how their daily contribution fits into the overall competitive plan. Conversely, organizations that have fallen behind tend to focus on all the internal issues that put them in a losing position. They typically engage in cost-reduction measures, and discredit those perceived to be re-

"Suddenly, one organization chooses to make a significant move to change the way they practice by rapidly adopting an EHR, leaving their competitors behind."

sponsible for the deteriorating performance. These are the companies that continually seek the quick fix.

> "Our research supports the notion that a breakaway is initiated when organizations decide to invest not just in technology, but in the people, processes and outcomes that can truly change healthcare."

Our research supports the notion that a breakaway is initiated when organizations decide to invest not just in technology, but in the people, processes and outcomes that can truly change healthcare. Technology alone does not solve problems, but with the right investment in people and processes, it can drive change. HIT has made significant progress in recent years through the HITECH Act and other legislation designed to create a sense of urgency. We now find ourselves closer than ever to achieving a higher level of patient care, quality and safety through technology. Now is our opportunity to make a bold move forward.

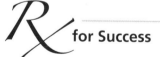 **for Success**

- Come to terms with the stress related to the adoption of an EHR and recognize that it will create a stronger and more resilient solution.
- Take advantage of the undeniable financial and clinical incentives of adopting an EHR today.
- Reap the benefits of a secure, standardized and shared EHR.
- Break away from competitors by adopting an EHR.

Why Implementation Is Not Adoption

Chapter Preview:

- Implementation and adoption of an EHR are not synonymous. To achieve improved outcomes, adoption is mandatory.

- Moving from an EHR implementation focus to an EHR adoption focus requires a significant overhaul in how we think, how we lead, and how we behave.

- Our research presents a methodology for lasting EHR adoption.

"*The innovation-decision process can lead to either adoption, **a decision to make full use of an innovation** as the best course of action available, or rejection, a decision not to adopt an innovation.*"

~ Everett M. Rogers

Diffusion of Innovations, 5th Ed., 1995

I t was 8 pm on a Friday evening, and the administrator of a 12-provider primary care practice sighed heavily as he reflected on the past six months. Their group had completed two successful go-live events in less than three months. By the end of the first quarter, each ambulatory site was running an EHR. Although it had not been pain-free, he felt like the implementation had gone smoothly. They had been strategic in choosing a vendor, involved the right staff in the application build, offered training to staff, and provided a great deal of support through go-live.

Today, only three months later, it felt like the entire project was spiraling out of control. Providers were frustrated by the time required to enter information, and several had even threatened to leave. A system audit indicated that clinicians were sharing generic user names and passwords; several nurses had documented potentially life-threatening errors they felt resulted from improper use of the new system; and to top it off, the upcoming executive committee meeting expected a presentation on expected outcomes from the EHR.

How does a successful implementation result in poor adoption? Easily! When decision-makers focus on just one event, a successful go-live, it is very easy to forego the processes that ensure adoption. Too many organizational leaders still believe that once the application goes live, users will embrace it. However, it is strikingly obvious after a go-live when the key elements of adoption have been left out. Many organizations have implemented an EHR, but very few have successfully adopted the EHR.

Implementation and adoption of an EHR are not synonymous. To achieve improved outcomes, adoption is mandatory

The terms *implementation* and *adoption* are often used interchangeably, but the outcomes from them are very different. Research suggests that implementation happens as soon as the application becomes available, but that adoption happens when the organization is using the application for clinical benefit (Jha et al, 2006). Another publication suggests that implementation happens when the organization "possesses" the application, while adoption happens when they actually use it (Florida Medical Quality Assurance Physician Practice Project, 2005-2008). Because it is critical to understand how organizations fail at EHR adoption, we will take this concept one step further.

Implementation happens when the EHR goes live, essentially after a successful switch "on" of the application. Adoption is a dynamic process that requires a sustained effort for the life of the application. A good indicator of a high level of adoption is when everyone is using the EHR according to the organization's prescribed policies and procedures, or best practices. Adoption enables an organization to achieve the outcomes

> "Implementation happens when the EHR goes live, essentially after a successful switch "on" of the application. Adoption is a dynamic process that requires a sustained effort for the life of the application"

described in the literature: improved quality, safety and efficiency, and ultimately a positive return on investment.

We first recognized the differences in outcomes between organizations that focus on implementation and those that focus on adoption as a result of our research and experience working with large national and regional healthcare organizations. We learned that the gap between perceived adoption of an EHR and actual use of the application is more common than we expected and is often overlooked as the organization struggles to understand the mediocre (and sometimes poor) outcomes from their EHR implementation.

Our experience and research has helped us understand the key differences between implementation and adoption. The following are indicators that adoption is at risk:

- Those charged with the implementation have a singular focus on the go-live event
- Information Technology (IT) executive is the primary owner of the EHR project
- Lack of a clearly-defined governance structure to sustain the EHR
- Disengaged leadership; leaders view the effort as compulsory rather than transformational
- Clinicians are rarely involved or are resistant, especially those in formal and informal leadership roles
- An institutional belief that implementation or go-live is the final step in the process

37

• No sustainable strategy to educate and engage end users to utilize the new workflow effectively
• Lack of metrics to assess adoption and ultimately achieve projected clinical and financial outcomes
• Lack of planning for post go-live workflow changes, end-user education, metrics, and overall optimization

Moving from an EHR implementation focus to an EHR adoption focus requires a significant overhaul in how we think, how we lead, and how we behave. Figure 3.1 illustrates the fundamental differences in how leaders approach a project-based implementation versus adoption. Adoption is a dynamic process focused on outcomes. When clinicians make the system their own, the reasons for utilizing the EHR outweigh the reasons to resist it. Quality of care, safety and other important clinical metrics become considerably more important than the project schedule and go-live activities. Additionally, this clinical ownership allows an executive to focus on the business issues and financial metrics. These changes "at the top" influence end-user attitude and the value of investing in educating. It also ensures that sustainment is not left to chance; it is a primary focus of the overall effort because the clinical and financial outcomes depend on it.

> **"Moving from an EHR implementation focus to an EHR adoption focus requires a significant overhaul in how we think, how we lead, and how we behave."**

Figure 3.1: Implementation vs. Adoption™

	Implementation	Adoption
Emphasis	Go-live (Event)	Outcomes (Process)
Ownership	Technical/ IT	Clinical/ Executive
Success Criteria	Technological Integrity	Role-based performance
Management Focus	Project Milestones & Cost	Quality of Care
Workflow Expectations	Repair	Redesign
Clinical Involvement	Negligible	Critical
End User Attitude	Apathetic or prejudiced	Adaptable
Metrics	Project Milestones	Outcomes
Training design	Demonstrate feature & function	Role-based Simulation, task completion
Sustainment post Go-live	Left to Chance	Primary Management Focus

Our primary argument that implementation is not adoption grew out of our research, as did the solution for lasting adoption. The adoption of an EHR is highly dependent on four components: engaged leadership, proficient end users, measurement of clinical and financial outcomes, and a plan to sustain the effort for the life of the application. The components can be illustrated in a simple graphic that represents the four corners of adoption (see Figure 3.2). Although we like the simplicity of this diagram, it does not really do the model justice. As we continue into the next four chapters, we build the model, illustrate how it operates, and demonstrate

> "The adoption of an EHR is highly dependent on four components: engaged leadership, proficient end users, measurement of clinical and financial outcomes, and a plan to sustain the effort for the life of the application."

how the components integrate to form a real solution to the problem of adoption.

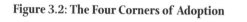

Figure 3.2: The Four Corners of Adoption

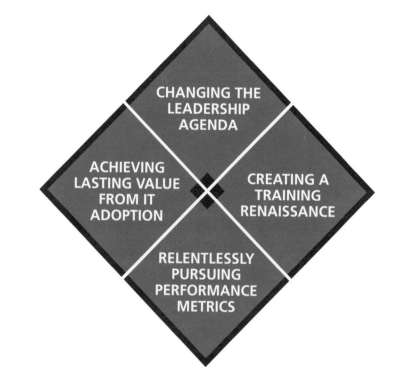

Moving from an EHR implementation focus to an EHR adoption focus requires a significant overhaul in how we think, how we lead, and how we behave

The challenges of EHR adoption are enormous and span the entire organization. The solutions to the problems of adoption are not immediately obvious and often eluded us during our original research. It was not until we were introduced to a science known as systems thinking that we began to mold a solution consistent with the ongoing and changing needs of healthcare.

In 1994, Peter Senge, a professor at MIT's Sloan School of Management, published *The Fifth Discipline*. Almost overnight, the book became a best seller, and Senge became famous for popularizing a science known as *systems thinking*. Systems thinking can help with the analysis of complex organizational problems, such as the adoption of an EHR. It is fundamentally different from traditional forms of analysis because it recognizes an inherent delay between cause and effect. Traditional event-based analysis assumes little or no delay between an event and its outcome, with the event itself scrutinized for success or failure. Event-based analysis also creates the impulse to identify the one or two issues that created a problem during the event and to direct a solution at the seemingly obvious cause.

To understand how systems thinking can help with the problem of adoption, we need to cover a few fundamentals. First of all, a *reinforcing feedback process* results in either a positive or negative acceleration of growth, and can be diagrammed as an archetype (Senge, 1994). An archetype is simply a diagram that tells a story. In Figure 3.3, the diagram for a *positive reinforcing process* is straightforward: consider the positive effect of beginning an exercise program and the improved mental and physical health that drives increased energy and reinforces exercise on subsequent days. Contrast this in Figure 3.4 with the effect of skipping one or more workouts, then feeling less fit and having less energy, resulting in skipping more workouts. This describes a *negative reinforcing process*.

Figure 3.3: The Positive Reinforcing Process of Exercise

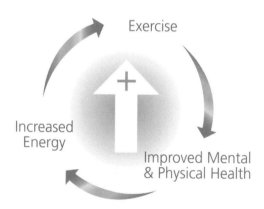

Figure 3.4: The Negative Reinforcing Process of Exercise

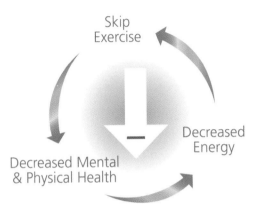

Many feedback processes contain delays between actions and their consequences (Senge, 1994). For example, it takes approximately 20 minutes for our stomachs to relay messages to our brains that we are full. When we are very hungry, we tend to eat so quickly that we completely overshoot the "full" response and end up feeling "stuffed." The inevitable delay between cause and effect in this feedback process leads us to overeat.

In relation to EHR adoption, feedback process delays may cause us to react with quick fixes that magnify the problem. Too often, we react to the problem of EHR adoption by coming up with solutions that only address the symptoms of the problem, leaving the problem itself unchanged or even worse. "Solutions that address only the symptoms of a problem, not the fundamental causes, tend to have short-term benefits at best" (Senge, 1994). Provider resistance, errors and security breaches are all symptoms of the bigger problem. If the problem is poor end-user adoption of the EHR, quick-fix solutions will not be effective. Quick fixes such as blaming providers, vendors or leaders, purchasing a new or upgraded application, forcing user compliance and ignoring poor outcomes also bring unintended consequences that actually cause a negative reinforcing feedback process, further delaying the solution of the problem. Identifying the root problems and employing sustainable solutions is the only way out of the quick-fix cycle. We will illustrate how the key drivers of adoption work together as a system using archetypes.

44

Our research represents a methodology for lasting EHR adoption

Based on the findings of our research, we developed a model that represents the four critical components of EHR adoption and how they work together. The diagram in Figure 3.5 uses Senge's approach to explain the interaction among the components of the model for EHR adoption. The foundation of sustainable adoption is engaged leadership, which sits at the center of the model. Developing a strategy for long-term adoption and establishing governance begins with engaged leadership. Engaged leadership makes or breaks the entire effort. As our research has shown, the second driver is an effective education and training program that results in proficient end users. Proficient clinicians and staff are a result of engaged leaders, so the model builds to the right of engaged leaders. Engaged leaders and proficient users produce desired clinical and financial outcomes, and they ensure the sustainment of these outcomes long-term. The sustainment loop is a balancing loop, which is a

"Based on the findings of our research, we developed a model that represents the four critical components of EHR adoption and how they work together."

critical component of the model because it ensures that the three reinforcing loops continue to move in a positive direction. Metrics serve as the "vital signs" for adoption over time, which reinforces the work being done by leaders and end users. In the next four chapters, we will dissect the model and take a deep dive into each of these areas to demonstrate how they integrate into a sustainable solution for EHR adoption.

45

Figure 3.5: Sustainable Solution to EHR Adoption

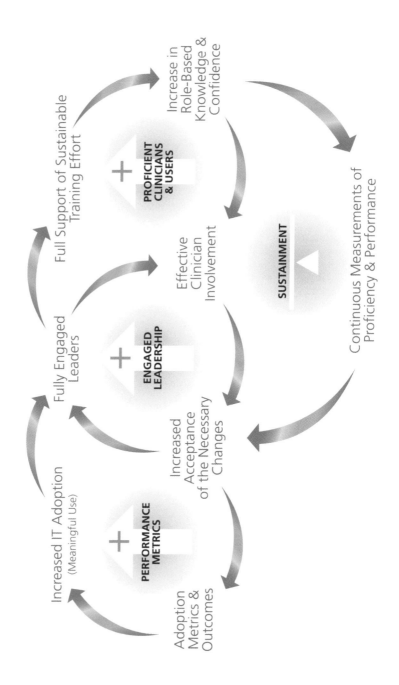

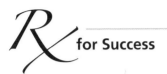

for Success

- Change your thinking regarding adoption to move beyond go-live myopia.
- Find a way to articulate the difference between implementation and adoption.
- Consider the long-term consequences of your decisions. Specifically resist quick-fix decisions that won't lead to end-user adoption.
- Find the courage to end the focus on implementation and to begin a journey toward adoption.

47

48

Changing the Leadership Agenda

Chapter Preview: A new leadership agenda focused on
leading EHR adoption:
- Develop a Stop Doing List
- Create a Tone at the Top in the
  organization
- Connect to the clinical leadership
- Empower the decision makers and
  define their sphere of influence

" *"What you do speaks so loud that I cannot hear what you say."* **"**

~ Ralph Waldo Emerson

Remembered for leading the Transcendentalist

movement of the early 19th century

The CEO of a mid-sized hospital is reviewing a recent assessment of the progress made one year after her organization's "big bang" go-live on clinical applications across acute and ambulatory care settings. Seated around a mahogany table are the members of the executive team, each sharing their thoughts about the organization's progress since replacing their legacy EHR system. The CIO and CMIO comment on the level of "change fatigue" throughout the organization. The CEO comments on the gross underestimation of the time and resource commitment to date. She is quick to add that the outcomes from the implementation work so far are mediocre, considering the time and resources invested. The executive team continues to address end-user resistance, workarounds, workflow discrepancies, patient safety concerns and resource shortages, to name a few. The effort has been exhausting at times, but they are finally beginning to see indicators of the metrics they expected from the new systems.

"Going into this, I did know how much work it would take," says the CEO. "I can't speak for others, but I honestly thought this was a project that would end after go-live. I knew the importance of leadership at the beginning, but I can't say I truly appreciated the effort required after that."

Although executives are becoming more aware of the critical role leadership plays in achieving clinical outcomes from technology, many also underestimate the continued level of engagement needed to sustain the application over the long-term.

Leadership's responsibility to drive EHR adoption continues long after the implementation. It requires an already overworked executive team to make adoption a daily priority. Effective leadership is the most fundamental and significant driver of adoption.

There is no greater barrier to adoption of a complex IT application in an ever-changing healthcare environment than believing we can simply pile this effort on top of all the other priorities and expect that we will be successful. Organizations that have disconnected, part-time and/or overworked leaders at the helm of an EHR effort will often struggle and may never fully adopt it. In contrast, organizations with leaders who are fully invested in the daily march toward adoption will not only reach the early stages of adoption, but will enjoy meaningful clinical and financial outcomes. To succeed in moving the people of an organization toward adoption of an EHR, leaders must change the way they previously approached implementations. The first priority must be to establish a new leadership agenda, which will create a reinforcing set of behaviors that begin the movement toward end-user adoption.

> **"There is no greater barrier to adoption of a complex IT application in an ever-changing healthcare environment than believing we can simply pile this effort on top of all the other priorities and expect that we will be successful."**

As we discussed in Chapter 3, leadership holds the central position of our model for lasting adoption. Leaders are in a critical position because they drive the system into either a positive or negative direction. More importantly, leaders need to be fully engaged over a significant period of time to maintain a positive reinforcing loop. Figure 4.1 illustrates how engaged leaders ensure clinician involvement and ultimately drive increased acceptance of the changes necessary for EHR adoption.

"The first priority must be to establish a new leadership agenda, which will create a reinforcing set of behaviors that begin the movement toward end-user adoption."

Figure 4.1: Adoption Model - Engaged Leadership

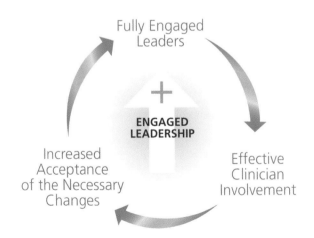

We carefully chose the term *engaged* to best describe the actions and behaviors required of leaders, and to avoid the negative connotation often associated with the term *change management*. Figure 4.2 illustrates a word map of terms related to the term engaged; interestingly, these terms also represent how engaged leaders describe their behavior on any given day as they interact with people, establish priorities and make decisions (THINKMAP Visual Thesaurus, 2016). It is engaged leaders who choose to see their roles and priorities differently and who ultimately lead their organizations successfully through change.

Figure 4.2: Word Map for the Term "Engaged"

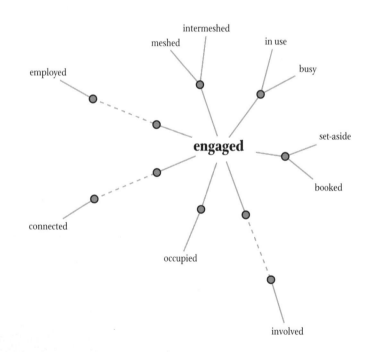

• • • Develop a Stop Doing List • • •

As stated earlier, the greatest barrier to adopting a complex IT application in an ever-changing healthcare environment is the belief that we can successfully heap this effort onto a long list of other priorities. Establishing a new leadership agenda requires freeing up time for those leading the effort. Without reprioritizing leaders' daily actions, all other actions are subject to inadequate time and attention. Jim Collins, the author of *Good to Great*, popularized the concept of the Stop Doing List. In his book, he contends that one of the commonalities of companies who are able to propel themselves from being just good to being great is that they examined everything they were currently doing and then consciously decided to stop working on some things, even some major things. In an interview with *TIME Magazine*, he is even more aggressive on this topic, arguing that many companies that have failed have done so because they simply had too many strategic initiatives in play (James, 2009). His book, *How the Mighty Fall*, centers on this topic. He contends that these initiatives literally choke an organization's growth due to lackluster performance in many areas and stellar performance in none.

"Leaders currently in charge of EHR adoption need to develop a ferocious understanding of what they are going to stop doing, and then maintain the courage to follow through on their decision."

Leaders currently in charge of EHR adoption need to develop

a ferocious understanding of what they are going to stop doing, and then maintain the courage to follow through on their decision. Because it demonstrates active commitment to end users who are affected by the new workflows, this may be the single greatest action toward successful adoption of an EHR.

Recall the example of HealthSouth from Chapter 1. As new hospitals continue to undergo implementations, HealthSouth requires all of its CEOs to study the factors that drive technology adoption and attend a CEO Forum designed to educate leaders on the effective strategies and priorities that ensure adoption. After a few pilot implementations, HealthSouth views its focus on leadership education and engagement as essential. The organization has learned the importance of creating an organization of engaged leaders who understand the fundamental activities that improve adoption, and it continues to serve as a pioneer in its steadfast commitment to make leadership engagement a priority in the overall effort.

Even though we cannot prescribe specific changes to leaders' priorities, we have identified some rules based on our experience with those who have succeeded:

1. Time is one of the most valuable resources among leadership and providers. Identify the most time-consuming projects and prioritize them using the following criteria:
   • Projects/meetings that do not directly affect quality of care or safety

- Projects/meetings that are not related to compliance or legal risk
- Projects that can be delayed with little overall impact
- Meetings that can be eliminated or consolidated

2. Be courageous: stop doing or postpone enough projects to enable the leadership team to declare EHR adoption as one of their top three priorities.

3. Openly communicate decisions to delay other projects throughout the organization. This provides the foundational message from leadership that EHR adoption is critical to the organization's mission. We have witnessed celebration, disbelief and clinicians' open arms when this has been done well.

4. Identify a governance method to ensure that new initiatives do not creep back into the list of priorities and consume the precious new time. We have seen great progress in stopping projects and meetings, only to find new projects and meetings sneaking in to take their place.

Create a Tone at the Top
of the organization

One of the most challenging aspects of leading the adoption of an EHR is transforming the project into a compelling and meaningful effort for everyone in the organization. When people, especially providers, believe in the cause, they will go to extraordinary lengths to ensure a successful outcome. This transformation creates and reinforces their commitment to the long-term goals of the effort.

Creating a message with purpose and constancy is not easy, and sustaining the message is even more difficult. When leaders create a tone that permeates the EHR adoption message, it will often overcome the imperfect delivery of messages shared among end users, helping to maintain the momentum behind the effort.

In a conversation with pianist, composer and recording artist Kevin Asbjörnson, he described the difference between a piano's *tune* and *tone* (Asbjörnson, 2008). We can draw an analogy from having multiple leaders tell the EHR adoption story. Tuning is the adjustment of a piano's strings to the correct pitch, ensuring notes played in octaves or chords will sound in harmony. Tuning is the organizational equivalent of how we connect people with equipment and workflow. By contrast, the quality of the sound

> "One of the most challenging aspects of leading the adoption of an EHR is transforming the project into a compelling and meaningful effort for everyone in the organization."

comes from adjusting the piano's tone. When the piano's tone is matched with the passion of the pianist, pure music radiates from the instrument.

Telling a powerful story of transformation through EHR adoption is the pure music that helps employees support the effort by addressing their biggest concerns. When leaders answer the big questions, like how the adoption of an EHR advances the mission of the organization, or how the changes will directly affect end users, employees are more likely to respond positively. The ultimate impact from the tone depends on providing compelling answers to these questions, but also on leader willingness and ability to make the message personal and transparent as they engage in dialogue about the changes. We have seen this effort unlock significant energy within those originally ambivalent about the effort.

There are myriad ways to develop the music from the leaders of the organization. The technique below represents a framework to develop the tone so that it resonates for years to come:

- The "Tone at the Top" requires a rigor similar to a marketing effort replete with a value proposition that connects to the mission of the organization.

- As with any respectable marketing program, a "brand" should be developed that delivers a symbolic moniker with lasting recognition for the adoption life cycle. Remember: this is a process that needs definition, not just an event.

- Keep in mind that the "tone" requires a constant rhythm from the leaders of the organization, and rhythm comes from a tempo of planned activities and communication efforts.

- Leaders must be visible and able to articulate the value proposition at any moment. Authenticity is the key ingredient in the message. Rather than creating new meetings, find a way to tap into current assemblies and gatherings.
- Build the "tone" into current employee feedback systems – or create a new one. Getting planned and periodic feedback from a cross-functional representation of the staff is part of the overall process to maintain the rhythm. Be prepared to modify the process if the message is not making an impact.

Connect to the clinical leadership

Provider adoption of the EHR is critical to an organization for four reasons:

1. Providers choose to bring their patients to the organization, often in preference to a competitor.
2. Providers personally provide and direct patient care, thus driving revenue and cost.
3. Providers are influential with colleagues and staff because of the informal organizational power derived from their medical knowledge and expertise, and from the trust and respect they are afforded.
4. Providers can be strong supporters or detractors of the EHR through the subtle exercise of this power.

The key to provider adoption is provider engagement. This engagement must occur at several levels. The first is at the governance level, through a provider body or council. A charter should formally establish the council, delineating the membership and often including representatives from all clinical departments. It is important to include EHR supporters as well as "curmudgeons." In most cases, the council chair should be a practicing provider and the CIO and CMO/CMIO should be staff to the council. The council should construct a vision statement that describes the benefits the EHR will provide to patients, providers, staff and the organization. The responsibilities and accountabilities of the council should be clearly explained in the charter; these often include specific policies, procedures and best practices for provider use of the EHR. Finally, and most importantly, the top leadership of the organization must formally endorse and empower the council to carry out its responsibilities.

The next levels of engagement are at the individual provider level. The council members should act as advocates for the EHR with their departmental colleagues. It can be very helpful to have several provider champions — individuals who are widely respected and well-connected within the organization. They do not have to be technology "nerds," and they often benefit from having at least a sprinkling of gray hair. Provider super users who are highly proficient in the use of the EHR can be valuable resources as at-the-elbow support for their colleagues and as mentors for new providers.

A high level of provider engagement can overcome or ameliorate the common barriers to provider adoption, including resistance to abandoning an existing EHR system, the investment

> "A high level of provider engagement can overcome or ameliorate the common barriers to provider adoption, including resistance to abandoning an existing EHR system, the investment of time required to learn the new system and the initial drop in productivity until the user attains proficiency."

of time required to learn the new system and the initial drop in productivity until the user attains proficiency.

Since writing the first edition of *Beyond Implementation*, a noteworthy trend has occurred nationwide. Decisions around clinical information systems are occurring jointly between the CIO and CMO/CMIO. CIOs, who were once the primary owners and leaders of EHR implementations, are sharing this responsibility with clinical leadership. CIOs play a key role in technology strategy and leading the change; however, CMOs and CMIOs are now leading the initiatives which impact clinical care, communicating with clinicians and promoting ongoing end-user participation, involvement, and engagement. This represents significant progress organizationally, as providers and nurses have the clinical expertise to direct and lead the effort to effectively achieve adoption.

Empower the decision makers and define their sphere of influence

Implementing an EHR requires thoughtful consideration of

the policies and procedures that will govern the use of the system. There are many stakeholders with a myriad of opinions and often competing interests that can dramatically slow adoption of the EHR. Adherence to a well-defined governance process ensures that the right people are involved at the right time with the right information. The lack of governance allows the wrong people to debate decisions endlessly, ignore standards easily and often conclude by making the wrong decisions. Leaders must establish strong governance processes to define expectations around adoption of the new application, involve the right stakeholders to make decisions, establish policies and best practices and ultimately evaluate performance against expectations. Governance should also be flexible enough to evolve over time. The governance needed during an implementation may be very different from the governance needed two years after go-live. In our experience, very few organizations appreciate the significance of governance in the adoption of an EHR.

Most organizations develop policies, procedures and best practices, but rarely measure their usage.

> "Effective governance closes the loop by monitoring adoption in the actual end-user work product. This creates a dynamic process that is able to evolve over time to meet the organization's needs."

We have all worked in organizations where significant time is spent on establishing best practices, only to find very few people actually observing them. This lack of accountability weakens the governance process. Effective governance closes the loop by monitoring adoption in the actual end-user work product. This creates a dynamic process that is able to evolve over time to meet the organization's needs.

Relentlessly pursue meaningful clinical and financial impact

The payoff for adopting an EHR comes in the form of clinical and financial outcomes. If results are neither tracked nor realized, the effort is truly a waste of time and money. Our expectations need to be realistic, but ultimately it is an organization's leaders who are accountable for relentlessly pursuing the tracking of outcomes.

When we conducted the interviews for our research, we were shocked at the lack of clinical and financial metrics being collected, especially considering the effort and money invested. In most cases, tracking metrics was simply not a high priority. The data were available, but the process for collecting, analyzing and reporting on the data was missing. The time and resources were not spent to obtain the story that the data could tell.

> **"If results are neither tracked nor realized, the effort is truly a waste of time and money."**

Since most people would agree that outcomes are critical to gauging the success of an EHR adoption, measurement of those outcomes must become part of the new leadership agenda. Leaders must incent the right people to collect, analyze and report on the data. Similar to engaging clinicians, this takes some finesse. The good news is that clinicians are generally interested in these metrics and may be more compliant with EHR use if they understand the clinical and financial goals. We usually suggest identifying a few key metrics that are easy to collect and that are of interest to the clinicians. Once those metrics are published, it does not take long to find the data enthusiasts in the organization and engage them in more sophisticated reporting. These metrics are the key to optimizing use of the system, achieving highly-engaged end users, and ultimately improving patient care.

The new leadership agenda for EHR adoption requires a significant change in how we lead. Newton's First Law of Motion states, "An object at rest tends to stay at rest and an object in motion tends to stay in motion with the same speed and in the same direction, *unless acted upon by an unbalanced force.*" This is an important concept to consider as we ask clinicians to change the way they practice medicine. We all have strong tendencies to keep doing what we're doing. In fact, it is our natural tendency to resist changes. In physics, this tendency to resist changes is called *inertia*. In healthcare, inertia represents the status quo. EHR adoption represents a significant change to the way we work, and it is natural to resist that change. However, because the benefits outweigh the pain of change in the

"In healthcare, that unbalanced force is engaged leaders who invest themselves in the outcome and create the momentum necessary for the organization to achieve adoption of an EHR."

65

long term, we need to find a way to overcome inertia. In physics, the only way to overcome inertia is to apply an unbalanced force. In healthcare, that unbalanced force is engaged leaders who invest themselves in the outcome and create the momentum necessary for the organization to achieve adoption of an EHR.

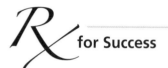 **for Success**

- Start today by establishing a new leadership agenda focused on EHR adoption.
- Develop a Stop Doing List that puts EHR adoption in the top three priorities.
- Create a Tone at the Top that permeates the entire organization.
- Engage and connect to clinical leadership to gain their support, which is critical for success.
- Empower the decision makers and clearly define their sphere of influence.
- Be relentless in the pursuit of meaningful clinical and financial outcomes.

CHAPTER FIVE

Creating a Training Renaissance

Chapter Preview:
- "The definition of insanity is doing the same thing over and over and expecting different results." – Benjamin Franklin
- Traditional training methods are a disservice to clinicians: they are slow, expensive and ineffective.
- We need a training renaissance to help clinicians learn new technology *fast*.
- Proficient and confident end users are the most valuable asset in achieving and maintaining adoption.

" *"The most important - and most vulnerable - connection between strategy and execution is the actual performance of people."*

~ Charles Fred

Breakaway

"The definition of insanity is doing the same thing over and over and expecting different results." – Benjamin Franklin

The road was jam-packed as car horns blared relentlessly in the stifling summer heat. We had just a few minutes before our meeting with the CIO of a healthcare system and we were still miles from our destination. Soon, the reason became apparent. Traffic signs reading "Parking" sprouted every quarter mile, and the police directing traffic pointed to the source of the problem: A prominent IT vendor was holding its first day of instructor-led training at the very place we were headed.

"You'd think a famous rock star was giving a concert. And on a weekday morning. This is madness," said our driver. With some luck and our driver's impressive knowledge of backroads, we finally arrived at our destination. Sweaty and out of breath, we apologized to the CIO, who looked just as frazzled.

"That's OK; believe me, I understand the disruption this is causing." He stood and glanced out the window at what appeared to be a large warehouse in the distance. "To think just last week I spent an entire afternoon trying to get porta potties for the new building we're renting. The plumbing doesn't work now, so I've had to scramble for a solution. I tell you, the whole thing is frustrating. Especially when it's already costing us $400,000 just to have the space for classroom training."

We didn't mention our experiences over the years. Hotel lobbies packed with luggage as hordes of consultants rushed to check in and out at the same time. Massive warehouses rented out to accommodate dozens of classroom sessions running simultaneously. School buses galore shuttling employees to offsite locations.

The CIO confessed that he didn't think his organization could logistically get all of its employees through the training. He wondered if there was a more sustainable and efficient means to educate end users on the enterprise application.

Traditional vendor training often follows this exact scenario, placing significant planning, logistical, and financial burdens on healthcare organizations. These difficulties transcend the executive level all the way into the classroom. Traditional training packs an unrealistic amount of content into marathon training sessions. Delays in the application build, testing and other unforeseen events often force training to take place at the last possible moment, then cramming as much material and information as possible into the available time period. The train-the-trainer method amplifies these problems; imagine depending on only a few people to transfer vital information to everyone in the organization - a recipe for disaster. Like the game of Telephone, information shared across multiple people loses integrity in each iteration. Train-the-trainer relies on individuals to understand, remember and clearly communicate complex information. All too often, inaccurate information is passed along instead. E-learning, web-based training and online learning provide consistent information, but they often simply repackage classroom instruction, which is rarely tailored to the learner's needs, and is subject to the same limitations of traditional training.

● ● ● Traditional training methods are a ● ● ● disservice to clinicians; they are slow, expensive and ineffective

When organizations struggle with adoption of new technology, they often blame the end user for resisting change. Complaints about provider resistance are especially common. While it is true that user resistance can slow adoption, the term places blame directly on users instead of addressing the real problem: how prepared for change is the organization, and how are users being educated? In truth, the user experience is simply a barometer of how well the organization has prepared participants for change and how effective the user education is. Provider resistance tends to be a symptom of poor training.

71

> "In truth, the user experience is simply a barometer of how prepared the organization is for change and how they have chosen to educate their users. Provider resistance is a symptom of poor training."

The term *speed-to-proficiency* describes our goal for end users. An effective learning process allows the organization to escape the endless cycle of repeating the same efforts while expecting different results. We want proficient end users who successfully and quickly learn exactly what they need to know in order to fulfill their specific role in the organization. Decision-makers who short-change training methods are three times more likely to have their IT projects fall short of business and project goals, and organizations that underfund training almost guarantee that end users will attain only a sub-standard understanding of new systems (Aldrich, 2000; Burleson, 2001; Wheatley, 2000). Compounding the problem, provider resistance is the most familiar complaint cited by organizations, while the most common provider response? "We don't have time for training and it isn't effective anyway!"

• • • We need a training renaissance to help • • • clinicians learn new technology *fast*

It is time to question the traditional training model for getting users up to speed on new technology. From nearly nine decades of research about adult learning, we know that humans do not learn without a natural progression from discovery through experience. The average human brain is a poor storage device for information and data, unless that information is recalled and

> "The one-time training event stuffed with an overloaded agenda is an almost certain waste if a user does not have the opportunity to progress through the natural learning process."

reinforced immediately through experiential activities. The one-time training event stuffed with an overloaded agenda is an almost certain waste if a user does not have the opportunity to progress through the natural learning process.

Adopting an EHR is an enormous undertaking for any organization, small or large, because it touches every employee and every operational process. In the past, healthcare organizations could spend days, weeks and months training and retraining staff. Today, there is a sense of urgency to adopt an EHR faster to improve clinical and financial outcomes. This requires a radically different process focused on helping clinicians achieve proficiency by role in the new technology quickly.

Adoption is driven by employing a sustainable and effective learning solution for clinicians and end users. Take a look at Figure 5.1. When the organization develops a curriculum focused on end-user knowledge and confidence, the outcome is proficiency. Proficiency among all users results in effective system use. To understand why high knowledge and confidence levels overcome provider resistance, consider how clinicians are traditionally trained in medicine. Providers have spent years honing their knowledge and experience in their fields of expertise. They are likely to resist because they are now being handed a tool they do not understand or trust to treat patients. When providers are highly knowl-

> "When providers are highly knowledgeable and confident in how to use the system to treat patients, they embrace the technology instead of resisting it."

edgeable and confident in how to use the system to treat patients, they embrace the technology instead of resisting it.

Figure 5.1: Adoption Model - Engaged Leadership, Proficient Clinicians & Users

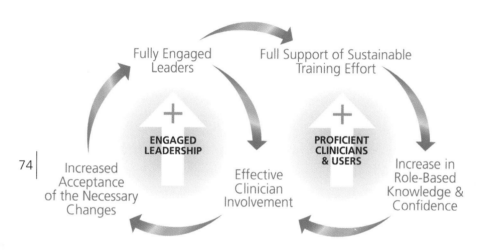

It is time to use this past century's research on human learning strategically, applying a heavy dose of common sense (Kolb, 1984). A number of steps and classifications have been used to describe the way in which a human learns and retains knowledge. We will use the aviation industry to introduce a new learning process and then apply these principles to healthcare.

In the early 1980s, the commercial airline industry faced a similar challenge to what we face in healthcare today. A breakthrough in manufacturing processes led to a dramatic decrease in the time it took to build an airplane. For the first time in history, the production of airplanes outpaced a pilot's ability to adopt the new digital avionics and flight control technology. It was a conundrum: the conversion of the new digital avionics from the outdated analog systems made air travel safer, but pilots could not get trained fast enough. Like a provider learning to use an EHR, pilots have received years of specialized training in their field; they have enormous responsibility for the safety of others, and they work in a complex and highly stressful environment. So why are we shocked when they refuse to attend classroom training or question the value of a train-the-trainer approach?

> "Just like pilots, clinicians must advance through four learning phases to learn the new information: introduction, assimilation, translation and accumulation (Fred, 2002)."

The commercial airline industry solved the problem by designing flight simulators that closely mimic the experience of flying an actual plane. They invented a solution that was relevant, timely, hands-on and sustainable – and that fit the pilot's needs.

Just like pilots, clinicians must advance through four learning phases to learn the new information: introduction, assimilation, translation and accumulation (Fred, 2002). In the first phase, the learner is exposed to a new set of data and recognizes that the information is different. In the second phase, the learner assimilates the new data with their own personal knowledge and experience. This is the stage in which the learner passes judgment on whether the new information or potential new skill has any benefit to them. When they perceive that it does not, their active participation in the learning process is at risk. In phase three, the learner places the new information into the context of their job, showing that they understand how it fits. Without translation available from a fourth phase, the learner stops at being informed and rarely makes the leap to any form of application or practice. Phases one, two and occasionally part of three are the usual fodder for the traditional training process. In fact, nearly 60 billion dollars per year are spent on this part of the proficiency process alone (American Society of Training and Development, 2009). Sadly, without the fourth phase, the end user cannot truly adopt, wasting both user time and organization resources.

> "Many organizations do not appreciate the importance of the users practicing what they have learned, testing through trial and error, and receiving feedback on their performance."

It is common for organizations to rely solely on the effectiveness of phases one and two; however, the highest payoff lies in the final and most time-consuming phase. In the fourth phase, knowledge is transformed into action through an accumulation of experiences using the new knowledge in practice or application. This phase is the most critical, yet is often left to chance when organizations plan an HIT implementation. Many organizations do not appreciate the importance of the users practicing what they have learned, testing through trial and error, and receiving feedback on their performance. As a result, organizations often leave this critical phase unfunded. Considered a cost savings in the short term, ignoring phase four actually costs the organization more because of increased turnover and overtime, clinician resistance to change and meager improvements to clinical outcomes. Organizations that employ phase four are able to shorten the cycle time to proficiency using rapid accumulation of experience, and affording the best opportunity to gain significant competitive advantage.

> "When designed correctly, simulators literally change how healthcare providers learn new technology."

When designed correctly, simulators literally change how healthcare providers learn new technology. First, they are designed separately for each role that uses the application. Providers and nurses do not perform the same tasks, so a generic simulator developed for only clinicians is ineffective. Traditional vendor training focuses on teaching individuals to learn how to use every function in an application, but individual users only need to learn the functions related to their specific roles. It is a mistake to teach every function of the entire application; it overwhelms the user with extraneous information and dilutes the information that is critical to their job role. For example, imagine if you were required to learn every function of Microsoft Excel before being able to create a simple spreadsheet. Most of us would much prefer to learn only the tasks necessary to create the spreadsheet, and then discover the bells and whistles later, if needed.

Consider a provider forced to attend three eight-hour EHR training sessions. He surely cannot help but question the level and depth of material planned for the week, not to mention the lost revenue from his not seeing patients on those days. He knows he will attend training along with medical students and residents – posing the challenge of how all the potential scenarios could possibly be covered. If they were all asked to achieve the same level of understanding of all of the material, most of the time spent in training would be wasted on at least two-thirds of the group. Common sense indicates that the target for proficiency varies greatly by role, because each role in healthcare varies so much. Someone in an administrative role does not require the medical proficiency of a nurse or provider. Clinicians require only the basics of how patients are arrived in the clinic, whereas front desk staff needs to know the most detail about scheduling, arrival, registration and check-out processes. One of the easiest, most pragmatic methods for reducing the cycle time to proficiency is to define a specific proficiency level required for a particular job role.

"The threshold level of proficiency is the point at which healthcare providers can collectively create and deliver value to a patient within a process (Fred, 2002)."

Defining the target proficiency level for performance in a particular assignment or task takes us on the shortest path to proficiency for a particular user or group of users. Beginning with the end in mind, we should always define the threshold level of proficiency before launching an elaborate system of training toward unnecessary goals.

The threshold level of proficiency is the point at which healthcare providers can collectively create and deliver value to a patient within a process (Fred, 2002).

The threshold level of proficiency is crucial to competitive advantage, because it is the point at which a user begins to contribute value to the operation in a particular job or task. For each of the varying degrees of contribution needed throughout an organization, there is a corresponding set of proficiency levels: discovery, literacy, fluency and mastery. Discovery, which combines the acquisition of new information with one's previous experience and knowledge, can be achieved through a formal training event, multiple forms of media, a dramatic event (e.g., safety accident) or through the grapevine. At the literacy level of proficiency, the learner can articulate newly-acquired information within the context of his or her job. Fluency is a function of the amount of experience accumulated over a period of time that allows someone to perform at an acceptable level. Mastery is also a function of the amount of experience accumulated over a period of time, but with enough experience gained to be considered a subject matter expert.

79

By identifying the required levels of proficiency across an organization, decision-makers take the first step toward a precise strategy that helps users adopt new technology. This helps them make the best use of both time and money to achieve crucial initial performance levels. When addressed this way, for the first time, proficiency is viewed across an organization strategically instead of tactically. With resources applied more strategically, workers begin reaching discovery and literacy levels very quickly. In addition, very few employees need to achieve mastery in their first learning efforts. Typically, only super users and IT (about five percent of the total group) need to reach the mastery level as their initial threshold. Providers, nurses, technicians, and administrative support employees all need varying levels of proficiency, but do not usually require mastery. The majority of the healthcare provider team only needs a fluency threshold level, and they can achieve this with a much shorter course, followed by rapid rounds of practice.

• • • Proficient and confident end users are • • • the most valuable asset in achieving and maintaining adoption

Software implementations often fail due to poor end-user adoption. The business case for a new EHR assumes that users will learn to use the system quickly. Yet end-user education is often underfunded, poorly planned and undervalued. When users cannot use the system according to prescribed workflows, the business case for the new system quickly falls apart, resulting in poor clinical and financial outcomes.

> **"Software implementations often fail due to poor end user adoption."**

Traditional training methods such as train-the-trainer and classroom instruction have never been truly effective ways for end users to acquire and apply knowledge. Classroom instruction is too passive a learning experience for the user. By the time the user

"Yet end-user education is often underfunded, poorly planned and undervalued."

gets their hands on the system, they typically cannot remember what they learned in class. Classroom training also takes clinicians and other critical staff away from work for hours or days. Train-the-trainer methods rely heavily on expert trainers, but these individuals often lack the time, knowledge and expertise to teach effectively on an individual level. Yet we know from our research and experience that many organizations still rely on these methods. Many also agree that their current training methods could be more effective, but most don't have the time, resources or staff to address the problem.

In a relatively short period, our industry has made significant advancements in health information technology. Through the efforts of the past few years, we now find ourselves capable of using health information systems to significantly improve clinical and financial outcomes. However, classroom training remains one of the largest barriers to progress. Even as organizations strive to improve outcomes through technology, many still apply this analog method to train their employees. So, while health information systems have the capability to improve outcomes, they are inhibited by obsolete processes that diminish their potential to achieve truly transformative and beneficial change.

Classroom training remains the status quo in the healthcare industry. It is embedded in the healthcare culture and has remained the safe choice for executive teams implementing multi-million dollar applications. To gain the most value from EHR systems, executives need a change in leadership thinking to initiate a cultural shift. While a seemingly insurmountable task, organizations such as HealthSouth (see Chapter 1) serve as fitting examples of the strategies and solutions required to depart from the paradigm of traditional training. Examples also exist across numerous other industries that have devalued classroom training and emphasized the importance of using technology to improve learning.

We had the opportunity to work with a large regional hospital in the process of replacing its existing EHR system. Our involvement began just as the organization had developed a plan to train providers and nurses on the new application before go-live. The organization had hired 16 trainers to deliver in-person instruction, requiring providers and nurses to attend 16 and 20 hours of classroom training, respectively. Faced with high costs to rent classroom space and cover floor shifts, and no way to truly sustain this model for the future, the organization's leadership team began considering other options. Our involvement in the process of educating the organization's end users came about through their realization that their existing training plan would last only 6 months and still require significant time and budgetary commitments. The accessibility, efficiency, repeatability, and consistency of our simulation-based education ultimately led the organization to ask for our help.

We began the new process by first engaging leadership and then developing a communication plan and an assertive marketing campaign to build an enthusiastic culture of adoption. We then developed project advisory and support teams with membership from all areas of the organization to ensure adequate representation and involvement in the final system release. We also performed extensive workflow analysis, capturing the current workflows and designing new workflows for each role in the organization. Users learned to perform the tasks for their role using online learning. Far from being a passive method of delivery, this online learning put the user inside simulations of real clinical scenarios. Users also solidified their knowledge and confidence through self-paced exercises designed to stretch their comprehension and learning retention. Individuals with expertise in the workflow by role then provided at-the-elbow support for other users. Providers received access to a private lounge for one-on-one coaching during specified hours of the day. Additionally, to accommodate highly complex or advanced material, we helped develop a limited number of instructor-led training sessions. The learning outcomes were dramatic. The average provider spent only seven and a half hours to complete their education, including practicing the key tasks in their role with the simulations. The average nurse spent only nine hours, including both simulation-based education and classroom training. Leading up to the go-live event, the organization's entire training schedule was reduced from six to two months, and provided significant time savings for all end users.

The pace at which learners adopt the new technology is critical, but so is the outcome of their learning. Knowledge and confidence are strong indicators of system proficiency. We developed a methodology for measuring both knowledge and confidence as indicators of proficiency. To evaluate proficiency, we assess end-user knowledge and confidence at baseline, after the application go-live, and regularly thereafter.

> "The pace at which learners adopt the new technology is critical, but so is the outcome of their learning."

After developing and deploying the education, we began collecting performance metrics. Our findings demonstrated significantly high course-completion scores, which is the first and best indicator of proficiency in the application. Among all hospital staff, 94 percent completed their required education, including 92 percent of providers. Additionally, we assessed end users by their ability to perform critical tasks in their workflow. Notably, all end users demonstrated significantly high rates of proficiency, with end users scoring on average 94 percent. Within days of the go-live event, our findings also showed that 73 percent of providers were using Computerized Provider Order Entry (CPOE) according to best practices. To drive continuous improvements and prevent erosion of these adoption results, organizations must sustain this level of knowledge and proficiency for their end users by continuing to review performance metrics. Changes to the application, new roles and responsibilities, workflow enhancements, turnover, and new hiring all threaten existing levels of end-user proficiency.

We also had the opportunity to work with one of the world's largest diagnostic imaging centers as they implemented a Radiology Information System/Picture Archiving and Communication System (RIS/PACS) for more than 870 end users at over 60 locations. Prior to our involvement, they had utilized a train-the-trainer model. Training consisted of eight to 12 hours of lecture and demonstration at an offsite location, in addition to travel time of two to four hours. After users at only a few sites completed training, it was apparent that the sites were not adopting the system. The organization documented the errors resulting from inconsistent practices and workarounds in the clinics. These errors resulted in increased insurance claim denials and delays, incorrect and incomplete patient information and increased days in accounts receivable. On average, it took employees 120 days (approximately 24 weeks, based on a five-day work week) to achieve fluency in the application. Again, the combination of these poor results led to our involvement and ultimately to an improved process for educating users.

Following our model for education and adoption, the average user became certified to use the application within four days. During the week of the go-live event, the average employee's time investment equaled approximately four days (two hours practicing with the simulators and four days using the application during go-live week). Therefore, the average speed to proficiency equaled four days, with the employees actually working in the live system for all but two hours. When compared to the initial site audits, the new process produced proficient users in four days, compared to 120 days, returning 116 days of productivity per employee to the organization. Extrapolated across all employees, the savings added up to an impressive 101,384 days (see Figure 5.2).

Figure 5.2: Train the Trainer Versus the Adoption Model

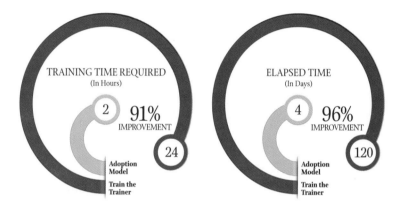

Our bias for metrics has served us well. We have accumulated data on over 1 million healthcare professionals who are actively engaged in the adoption process. Through our research and experience, we have established benchmarks for healthcare organizations striving to improve adoption of new healthcare technologies. Our research indicates that a minimum of 90 percent of users must complete their required education to demonstrate proficiency before the go-live event. We have also found that assessing user knowledge and confidence is a vital activity, because both measures are key indicators of proficiency and adoption of the application. At least 90 percent of end users must have either *excellent* or *good* levels of knowledge and confidence in using the new technology after the initial go-live. By the end of the first year, organizations should achieve at least 95 percent on both knowledge and confidence, and they should maintain that level for the lifetime of the application.

Today's IT vendors may require organizations to follow a "blended learning approach," which pairs classroom training with some form of online learning. Based on our research, however, the classroom is one of the least effective environments for teaching a user how to perform tasks in a new system. E-learning offers few advantages and several significant disadvantages for user engagement. We need to continue to innovate around the most effective experience that will allow users to gain the most value from these systems. The aerospace industry clearly demonstrated the value of a simulation-based approach that enables end users the freedom to accumulate experience in a safe and relevant environment. Learning must be relevant, easily digestible, consistent and specific to user workflow in order to produce the results we seek long past go-live. Give learners the opportunity to become proficient in the tasks they use to serve patients, and they will quickly adopt the new technology.

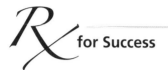
for Success

- Choose to train clinicians in a new way. The processes and technology exist to dramatically improve end-user adoption.
- Dedicate your training effort to ensuring that end users achieve threshold proficiency.
- Create an environment where end users can practice and accumulate experience in the application using clinical scenarios.
- Require that every end user achieve high levels of proficiency, knowledge and confidence.

Relentlessly Pursuing Performance Metrics

Chapter Preview:
- Adoption is a prerequisite for meaningful use and we must measure it.
- The first indicator of adoption is end-user proficiency.
- Performance metrics demonstrate the value of adoption through improved clinical and financial outcomes.
- Performance metrics drive the organization to optimize EHR use.

" *"Trying to improve something when you don't have a means of measurement and performance standards is like setting out on a cross-country trip in a car without a fuel gauge. You can make calculated guesses and assumptions based on experience and observations, but without hard data, conclusions are based on insufficient evidence."*

~ Mikel Harry
Six Sigma Author

The small conference room barely accommodated those in attendance, and the heated discussion was making the room feel smaller by the minute. "We already provide exceptional care to our patients. I am not convinced an EHR will change the quality of care we provide," declared a cardiologist. A primary care provider chimed in, "Our margins continue to erode as CMS cuts reimbursement; how can we afford this?" A well-respected provider spoke up next, "Productivity may drop as much as 50% after an EHR implementation. What are the plans to compensate us during that time?" These are just a few of the questions on providers' minds as they grapple with the changes coming their way. Providers and clinicians spend their days interpreting data from multiple sources and using that information to treat patients. Because they approach problems from an analytical perspective, metrics are one of the most persuasive tools for convincing providers of the benefits of an EHR accruing directly to their patients and to them. In addition to gaining provider buy-in, part of the reward of capturing performance metrics is using them to drive continuous improvements in clinical and financial outcomes. In this chapter, we will demonstrate how metrics facilitate provider buy-in, improved adoption and meaningful use of an EHR. We will also explore the value of conducting routine health checks of EHR adoption.

Adoption is a prerequisite for improving outcomes and we must measure it

Since writing the first edition of *Beyond Implementation*, legislation governing EHR use has changed. As discussed in Chapter 2, legislation like the Health Information Technology for Economic and Clinical Health (HITECH) Act is creating disruption across healthcare. However, in most cases, the legislation falls short of the vision and the value comes from the work done at the local level in healthcare organizations. It is worth noting that the HITECH Act, Physician Quality Reporting System (PQRS), and Medicare Access and Chip Reauthorization Act (MACRA) share the same purpose: to improve patient care and outcomes. Despite changes in penalties, incentives, and payment models, capturing performance metrics is vital to EHR adoption and to improving clinical and financial outcomes.

Adoption is a prerequisite for improved outcomes. A good indicator of a high level of adoption is when everyone is using the EHR according to the organization's prescribed policies and procedures, or best practices. No matter the legislation, organizations pursuing adoption must ensure the effort is directly aligned with the desire to improve clinical outcomes.

In Chapter Five, *Using Speed to Proficiency to Create a Training Renaissance*, we discussed an effective methodology to achieve end-user adoption - but following the methodology isn't enough. The only way to know that end users have actually adopted the EHR is to measure their progress. It is clear from our research that very few organizations are measuring adoption. Without measurement, the organization has only subjective assessments of adoption and no way to establish a plan for improvement. We recognize that 100 percent adoption may be unrealistic due to changes in workflow, staff turnover and upgrades, but organizations with the highest rates of adoption will certainly achieve the greatest return on their investment in both clinical and financial terms.

> **"The only way to know that end users have actually adopted the EHR is to measure their progress."**

The first indicator of adoption is end-user proficiency

How would most of us answer the question, "Are our end users proficient in the tasks required to use the EHR?" Many organizations assume their training and education will automatically produce end users with a high level of knowledge and confidence in their ability to use new technology, indicating proficiency in their role. But they don't measure the outcomes of their education and training programs. Measurement of outcomes is a critical step, but

> **"Forgoing measurement of end-user proficiency means passing on the chance to identify gaps in adoption and ultimately achieve improved clinical and financial outcomes."**

one that most organizations don't even consider. Forgoing measurement of end-user proficiency means passing on the chance to identify gaps in adoption and ultimately achieve improved clinical and financial outcomes. Proficiency is a key indicator of end users' ability to use new technology. If we forego the measurement of end-user proficiency, we lose the opportunity to identify gaps in adoption, which ultimately limits our ability to achieve improved clinical and financial outcomes.

Simulators are an excellent tool for teaching because they not only allow individuals to learn new information in the most effective way, but they also provide consistent information to all users. Additionally, they capture valuable data about users' ability to complete role-based tasks in the new system. Collecting data directly from simulators allows organizations to make improvements to education and training programs, and signals knowledge decay users commonly experience after a single training event. Organizations may also choose to grant access to the EHR only once a user tests at the required level of proficiency in the new application.

We also strongly believe that the combination of high knowledge and confidence produces lasting adoption. Employee confidence level is highly correlated with long-term adoption. Typically, when they are introduced to a new system, users rate their confidence level as either poor or fair. As their knowledge increases, their confidence begins to increase. In fact, confidence quickly becomes the driver for achieving higher levels of knowledge. Consider the use of a new technology, like a cell phone. Someone who decides to upgrade an archaic 2-year old phone to the latest and greatest, feature-rich cell phone quickly realizes that the tasks they mastered on the old phone function differently on the new phone. Knowledge is low and confidence is in the tank. By watching the demo feature on the new phone, the user's knowledge quickly improves, and soon the new phone's basic functions become easier to master. Newfound confidence actually fuels one's willingness to explore new functionality. The interplay between knowledge and confidence is something we all experience daily as we learn.

We recommend collecting baseline data for knowledge and confidence and measuring it again after go-live, and at regular intervals thereafter. Our data suggest that organizations should strive for 90 to 95 percent of end users falling in the *excellent* or *good* category for both knowledge and confidence. Once they achieve that milestone, it is time to examine performance metrics in terms of clinical and financial outcomes.

95

Performance metrics demonstrate the value of adoption through improved clinical and financial outcomes

The most challenging and valuable process is the measurement of *performance metrics*, valuable because these represent the clinical and financial outcomes that drive an organization to purchase an EHR. Collecting performance metrics is often a daunting task because organizations must customize measurements to represent their specific desired outcomes. Examples of these metrics can include increased adherence to clinical guidelines, increased revenue from improved accuracy in charge capture, reduction in transcription costs and increased RVUs per provider per month. These metrics, among others, will truly validate the investment in an EHR.

Figure 6.1 illustrates the role of performance metrics in the adoption model. Once we achieve a high level of end-user proficiency, the EHR data provides fertile ground for examining the clinical and financial outcomes. Performance metrics also reinforce the continued effort of keeping leaders engaged and maintaining our process for educating end users. As we discussed early in this chapter, metrics can also motivate end users to change their behavior. If they are used correctly, a dashboard of relevant and timely metrics becomes the focus of the EHR effort.

The first step is to identify the key performance metrics. Most organizations begin the EHR selection process with a formal justification for purchasing their EHR, often in the form of a business case. A strong business case identifies measurable critical outcomes from the EHR. To simplify the process, use research questions to formulate desired outcomes. For example, "Is the EHR reducing personnel, chart supplies and storage costs in the medical records department?"

Once performance metrics are identified, the real work begins: capturing the appropriate data. Unfortunately, most EHR vendors do not provide data reports with the level of detail required to track metrics. Designing a methodology for capturing the data required to address the key metrics is complex.

Figure 6.1: Adoption Model - Engaged Leadership, Proficient Clinicians & Users, Performance Metrics

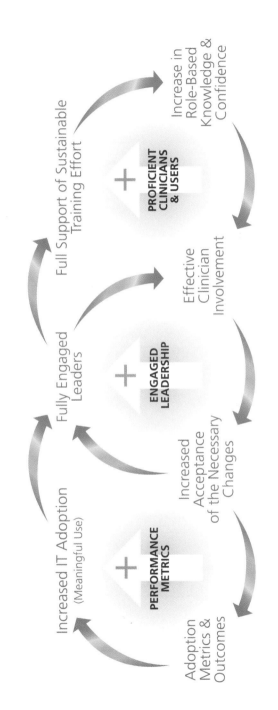

The expertise of a trained clinical researcher and often a statistician is very valuable in designing, analyzing and summarizing the data. The commitment to identify even just a few key metrics provides enormous value to the organization. First, it is very handy in proving meaningful use. Second, it can be used as a dashboard for measuring the performance of the EHR over the life of the application. Most importantly, it drives continual improvement in specific areas of value to the organization. It also creates the discipline needed to assess the value of all health information technology investments objectively.

Performance metrics drive the organization to optimize use of the EHR

Performance is naturally at risk of erosion over time. Part of the challenge for organizations is ensuring that the process of capturing performance metrics continues long-term, and that these data are used to make continuous improvements to the adoption of the EHR system. Our research shows that an effective solution is to conduct periodic assessments of application use. Just as routine health exams help prevent chronic diseases in patients, screenings of EHR adoption help avoid major negative consequences. By implementing frequent and ongoing evaluations of performance, healthcare organizations can identify problems in their infancy before they pose systemic or significant harm. Interviewing key decision-makers and influencers across the organization about the strengths and weaknesses of the application and areas of concern helps reveal underlying issues. By combining this information with quantitative data and observations of end users working in the system, the organization gains a timely and accurate reflection of the organization's current state of adoption.

> "Organizations that measure their performance and maintain the tenacity to continually improve will be rewarded with a stellar reputation, loyal employees and clinical and financial success."

Throughout our country, we can find examples of healthcare organizations at various stages of EHR adoption. Each has the opportunity to improve on key performance metrics. Organizations that measure their performance and maintain the tenacity to continually improve will be rewarded with a stellar reputation, loyal employees and clinical and financial success.

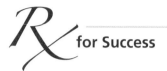
for Success

- Measure employee knowledge and confidence to gauge their level of proficiency.
- Develop a "dashboard" to consistently measure, analyze and communicate key clinical and financial outcomes.
- Commit to utilizing these performance metrics to identify areas of improvement and focus on solutions that actually improve adoption.
- Conduct routine health checks to evaluate the current state of adoption.

Achieving Lasting Value from IT Adoption

Chapter Preview:
- Most organizations grossly underestimate the effort and resources required to sustain IT adoption.
- Measurements of end-user adoption reliably predict improvements and regression in adoption.
- Resources, communications, education and metrics must be *shared, updated* and *easy to find* for the life of the application.

> **"** *"Sustainable transformations follow a predictable pattern of buildup and breakthrough."*

~ Jim Collins

From Good to Great

Several years ago, a reputable IT vendor offered us free use of their software. The software provided equipment monitoring that would be valuable to us. Initially, we were excited. The functionality aligned with our needs exactly, and the application was robust enough to grow with us. We had a need and the software fulfilled the need. The system served IT directly, so our Director of IT led the implementation and kept our senior management team updated on the progress. We couldn't wait to have access to the dashboard of data promised by the vendor. Months after the implementation, we were still waiting. Although the "free" price tag was alluring, we quickly recognized that the actual maintenance costs and labor required to make the application truly valuable to our organization were missing. This story drives home a concept that we all understand, but often overlook. Underestimating the "care and feeding" required to maintain a valuable investment puts the entire project at risk. It

> **"Underestimating the 'care and feeding' required to maintain a valuable investment puts the entire project at risk."**

sounds simple, but we all need to remember the importance of sustainability even when initially getting excited about the value of an investment. It is common to under-appreciate the effort it takes to maintain the value of something, even something that initially costs nothing.

Most organizations grossly underestimate the effort and resources required to sustain IT adoption

Let's consider the shift in thinking required to move from implementing an EHR to maintaining high levels of adoption over the life of the application. This is analogous to the shift required to sustain long-term weight maintenance after successful weight loss. The findings from a telehealth study are applicable here (Haugen, 2007). The percentage of overweight adults in the U.S. is staggering and continues to rise. Today, over 70 percent of adults in the United States are overweight (Centers for Disease Control, 2014) and 51 percent of Americans are actively trying to lose weight (Brown, 2013). But the problem isn't weight loss! Many of us have successfully lost weight, but can't keep the weight off. As a matter of fact, we regain all the weight (and often more) within 3-5 years (Wadden, 1993; Kramer, 1989). This isn't a complex concept: dieting doesn't incent long-term lifestyle change, thus the weight re-gain. As a result of the initial findings, an innovative program was developed to keep people engaged at various levels depending on their progression through the program. The researchers knew that people needed to practice weight management behaviors actively - for years, not months.

In the world of EHR adoption, we have taken the "dieting" approach to implementing new software solutions in our healthcare settings for too long. We prepare for a go-live event. After go-live, we fall back into our comfortable old habits - resulting in workarounds, regression to ineffective workflows, insufficient training for new users, poor communication and errors. The process of adoption requires a radically different discipline, and the real work begins at go-live.

> **"The process of adoption requires a radically different discipline, and the real work begins at go-live."**

After the successful implementation of a new technology, our tendency is to move on to the next project. We are often busy juggling multiple projects and it actually feels like a relief to move it off our list of highest priorities. A sustainment plan addresses two important areas. First, it establishes how the organization will support the ongoing needs of the end users for the life of the application. This includes communication, education and maintenance of materials and resources. Second, it establishes how and when metrics will be collected to assess end-user adoption and performance. Lack of planning and execution in these two areas will lead to a slow and steady deterioration in end-user adoption over time.

Effective sustainability plans require resources, time and money. Keep in mind that adoption is never static; it is continually either improving or degrading in the organization. Figure 7.1 illustrates the dynamic nature of adoption over the life cycle of an application. Drops in proficiency appear after upgrades or changes to the application. Leadership must plan for the investment and fund it if their ultimate goal is improved performance. Most organizations only achieve modest adoption after a go-live event, and it takes relentless focus to achieve the levels of adoption needed to improve quality of care, patient safety and financial outcomes. Sustainability plans are most successful when they are part of the initial budgeting and planning stages for an EHR.

Figure 7.1: The Life Cycle of Adoption

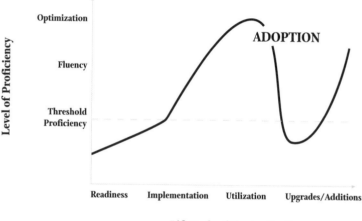

In our first edition of *Beyond Implementation*, we wrote about the University Clinical Health (UCH, formerly known as UT Medical Group) story, which represented the real struggles many organizations were experiencing as they navigated the journey of EHR adoption. Their experiences were consistent with our early research findings and the stories we continue to hear from healthcare leaders today. Since we first told their story, UCH's path to EHR adoption has presented new challenges and even some epic wins. They developed a rigor and focus on adoption that brought impressive outcomes. They understood the drivers of adoption which created real momentum for reaching the top third of the adoption curve in Figure 7.1. Like many other organizations we studied, they also saw erosion of adoption at times during their journey. The factors that caused UCH's adoption to erode were the same factors that are common to all organizations. It started with turnover in the organization's leadership team, which led to a decrease in engagement as new executives prioritized other activities. The organization also experienced significant changes to its EHR system and workflows that dramatically decreased end users' knowledge and confidence in the application, necessitating reeducation. Another challenge was employee turnover, which prompted the need for new rounds of hiring and onboarding, and temporarily resulted in decreased proficiency levels. Despite this valley in the adoption curve, UCH reengaged as a leadership team, reeducated its end users, leveraged performance metrics to drive continuous improvements, and committed to sustaining its efforts for the future. This is the dynamic nature of successful EHR adoption – it requires continual care and feeding. Today, UCH is once again experiencing high levels of adoption and provides a telling example of the importance and practicality of continuing this work.

Figure 7.2: Sustainable Solution to EHR Adoption

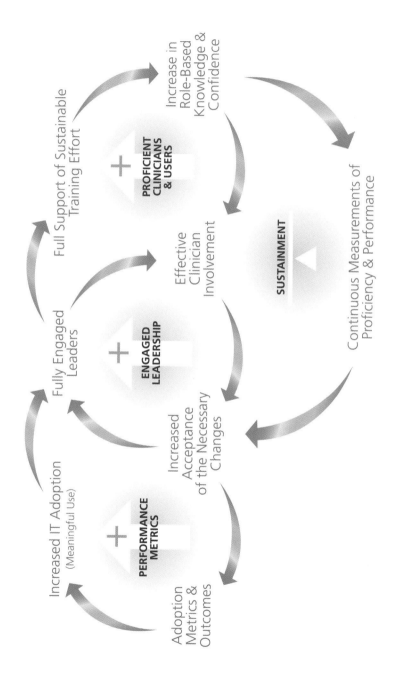

Measurements of end-user adoption reliably predict improvements and regression in adoption

Sustainment means more than simply maintaining the status quo. When sustainment becomes a passive process, it is a waste of resources. Metrics are the differentiating factor between a highly effective sustainment plan and a mediocre one. Knowledge and confidence metrics serve as a barometer for end-user proficiency level, providing the earliest indication of adoption, or use of the application according to the organization's best practices. Ultimately, performance metrics are powerful indicators of whether end users are improving, maintaining or regressing in their adoption of the system. If we get an early warning that proficiency is slipping, we can react quickly to address the problem. These metrics are the balancing force for the entire adoption model. As shown in Figure 7.2, this balancing loop that measures proficiency and performance ensures that all three of the reinforcing feedback loops continue in a positive direction. Remember, the reinforcing loops are always at risk of moving in the opposite direction and creating barriers or degradation of EHR adoption. Metrics act just as the scale does in long-term weight management; they are the

> "Ultimately, performance metrics are powerful indicators of whether end users are improving, maintaining or regressing in their adoption of the system."

first indicator that we are falling back into old behaviors that are not consistent with sustainable adoption.

Metrics also keep us on track when performance does not meet expectations. Let's consider two different scenarios to illustrate this idea. In both scenarios, the go-live event is successful, but specific performance metrics do not meet expectations. In most cases, the performance metrics are not achieved because the system is not being utilized effectively. This may be due to inadequate training and therefore lower proficiency, or a problem with the actual performance by end users in the system. Measuring end-user proficiency allows us to identify "pockets" of low proficiency among certain users or departments and make sure they receive the education needed. Once users are proficient, we can refocus our attention on the performance metrics. The second scenario is less common, but also more difficult to diagnose. Sometimes users are proficient, but specific performance metrics are still not meeting our expectations. In this case, we need to analyze the specific metric. Are we asking the right question? Are we collecting the right data? Are we examining a very small change or a rare occurrence? There may also be a delay in achieving certain metrics, especially if the measurements are examining small changes. A normal delay can wreak havoc if we start throwing quick fixes at the problem. In this situation, staying the course and having confidence in the metrics brings desired results.

Resilience, communications, education and metrics must be shared, updated and easy to find for the life of the application

Executives, managers and clinicians must continue to lead EHR adoption long after the initial implementation. This is a difficult task because of typical time and resource constraints in healthcare, but achieving the highest levels of adoption requires innovative, efficient and effective solutions to these common problems.

Our research indicates that the ability to achieve and sustain high adoption over time is impacted by turnover, staff growth, workflow changes, application updates and the human factors of individual learning and retention. How do we determine the funds and resources needed to overcome these factors? First, consider what the users need in order to maintain high levels of knowledge and confidence in using the EHR. Answering a series of questions can be effective in helping understand user needs:

- How can we effectively communicate updates and changes in workflow to the users?
- How do we educate new users?

> "Executives, managers and clinicians must continue to lead EHR adoption long after the initial implementation. This is a difficult task because of typical time and resource constraints in healthcare, but achieving the highest levels of adoption requires innovative, efficient and effective solutions to these common problems"

111

- How do we update quick reference guides or course materials?
- When are metrics collected and how are they used?

Second, consider the best approach for meeting these needs. Most organizations are already stretching their resources to the limit, and they assume more resources are required to achieve sustainment. Instead, they should consider how technology can be used to expand their reach within the organization.

Imagine a place dedicated to sustaining EHR adoption in the organization, uncluttered by every update, communication and document from every project; this place would focus solely on improving and sustaining the adoption of an EHR. It would encompass many tools, including a learning management system (LMS), document management and search capability, communication posts, the ability to plan and archive meetings, and much more.

"Imagine a place dedicated to sustaining EHR adoption in the organization, uncluttered by every update, communication and document from every project; this place would focus solely on improving and sustaining the adoption of an EHR."

Most importantly, end users would find it incredibly valuable: easy to access, relevant and meaningful.

Based on our work with healthcare clients who struggled with sustainment, we developed a place like this. We developed a solution that addresses many of the barriers to lasting adoption. We started by identifying the critical tools and resources required to meet the user needs and then we made it easy to access and use. The concept we created is a learning community that delivers value directly to end users.

The learning community concept is tool that ensures the four drivers of adoption can be easily managed and sustained over time. We share our ideas around this tool to give you a sense of what is possible and what its design may entail. Our ideas are by no means prescriptive or absolute; rather, they are based on the successful experiences of organizations that have completed this work. However, we recommend organizations develop some tools or approaches that facilitate and support each of the four drivers of adoption. For instance, the solution should enable leadership to communicate with end users, as well as govern and oversee their performance. It should also connect end users with their relevant education and track their performance for completion and possible remediation. These performance data should be available to individuals, supervisors, and leadership. And lastly, it should facilitate continued access to updates and resources to sustain performance through changes to the organization, application, and/or personnel.

Our community concept is an enterprise application that assists healthcare organizations with content and learning management. Based entirely online, it enables end users to access valuable resources, tools and activities as needed from work or at home, maximizing productivity and minimizing disruptions during peak hours. This application also houses all online courses or task-based simulators with the capabilities of a learning management system.

Task-based simulators help users become proficient in the tasks they must perform in the system, and they are updated regularly to reflect changes in workflow. This enterprise application tracks the completion of each course or simulator to measure whether end users have completed their required education. For evaluations, the application provides assessments that test end users' ability to complete tasks specific to their role and tracks performance throughout their workflow. This system makes completion and performance metrics available to individual end users, as well as to leadership and supervisors for governance and remediation. For those organizations that choose to offer classroom education, the application also eliminates logistical hurdles by enabling learners to view and enroll in sessions. Additionally, this enterprise system hosts a communication forum to facilitate timely updates, announcements, and discussions. Overall, the system takes complicated processes and tools and makes them easy to use. This approach offers significant advantages for overcoming the time and resource constraints many organizations feel around sustainability. It gives users access to timely, relevant and valuable information. It also eases the strain on resources, while still requiring a commitment to the care and feeding of each element in support of lasting end-user adoption. Like other factors that facilitate adoption, organizations must commit to sustain the enterprise system long-term to support end users through application upgrades, workflow enhancements, changes in roles and responsibilities, as well as to support and develop new hires.

The value of sustaining adoption is not limited to healthcare organizations. Our experiences have shown that vendors also benefit by having an engaged leadership team, offering accessible and repeatable education to employees, capturing performance metrics to drive continuous improvements, and sustaining applications long-term.

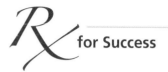

for Success

- Plan now for sustainment by committing appropriate resources, time and funds.
- Develop a reporting and analysis process to determine where to focus sustainment efforts.
- Find an innovative solution to expand the reach to end users. A web-based community is an example of a technology that gives users timely, relevant and valuable information.

CHAPTER EIGHT

The Journey Continues…

118

Adoption is not a destination, but a continuous journey. We don't arrive at adoption, but relentlessly pursue its rewards through a fierce and ongoing commitment to excellence. The journey is difficult, tiresome and necessary to achieve the expected outcomes. Now more than ever, we must make adoption a vital priority as our industry stands at the brink of truly transforming productivity, quality and safety through health information technology.

The title of *Beyond Implementation* has changed since the first edition. No longer do we use the acronym "EMR" to describe the type of adoption contained in these pages. That's because adoption is not limited to one type of clinical information system. Instead, the model we present suggests a universal process for any organization facing any disruptive change brought on by healthcare technology. For this reason, we have changed our title to broaden our scope, and we encourage organizations to apply our model to all of their projects.

Achieving and sustaining adoption requires four key areas of focus. The most important is leadership, which ignites the overall effort by engaging the collective organization on the path forward. From a leadership standpoint, setting the tone, establishing the vision, engaging clinical leadership and fostering end-user engagement are just a few of the many elements needed to drive successful adoption. Yet adoption is not complete without accessible, sustainable, scalable, and targeted means to get end users up to speed. End users need the knowledge, confidence, and proficiency to perform critical tasks in the live application, and simulation-based education affords the best model for EHR systems. The dynamic nature of adoption and the quest to improve care require another important element: performance metrics. Individuals, supervisors, and leadership need continual access to real-time data to take the pulse of how end users are performing relative to their roles and responsibilities. In turn, these performance metrics must be leveraged to drive continuous improvements. Adoption also requires the sustained and ongoing commitment to leadership, education, and performance metrics to overcome the tyranny of time and uncertainty of application upgrades or changes, workflow enhancements, turnover, changes in roles and responsibilities, and new hiring.

Through our research and experience with healthcare organizations, we learned several key lessons which offer value to any healthcare leader, professional, or innovator engaged in this work. Our first lesson came from our partnership with HealthSouth. As discussed in Chapter 1, HealthSouth demonstrated that adoption is only achievable through relentless commitment to the goal. The organization remained steadfast in its seemingly impossible vision of undergoing 98 implementations across all of its hospitals. After the first few implementations, the organization's leaders quickly realized that they could not sustain their current approach to EHR implementation if they wanted to meet the organization's goals. The organization made a bold commitment to reset and follow a new approach - an adoption approach - to realize its mission.

Through this struggle, HealthSouth emerged as a true innovator and a testament to adoption and serves as an example to every organization on how to best lead this important work.

In addition to HealthSouth's commitment to adoption, we also learned that organizations benefit from developing and applying strategies that support the four drivers of adoption. Due to its sheer size and the number of implementations it faced, HealthSouth developed a scalable, repeatable process for getting hospitals prepared for a quick and effective implementation. This demonstrates the value of organizations considering their unique strengths, weaknesses, opportunities and threats that may impact their adoption. While the four key drivers of adoption represent essential activities, organizations should also pursue other strategies that improve their ability to optimize the application.

Another lesson came from our work with MCHS. Up until then, we most often witnessed organizations waiting to begin their adoption work until the go-live event loomed, and then the challenges they faced as a result of their procrastination. Unlike these organizations, MCHS's leadership began generating awareness and end-user engagement in the project one year before the implementation. They also began discussions and planning around education, tracking performance metrics, and sustaining the overall effort, giving the organization ample time to prepare and invest in the initiative.

Our research also shows the value of conducting routine health checks as a supplemental activity to gathering quantitative data. While data pertaining to end-user knowledge, confidence and proficiency are vital, they don't tell the entire story. Conducting interviews with key decision-makers and influencers across the organization can help uncover underlying issues with the application itself or with how it's being used. Combining this information with quantitative data and in-person observations creates a comprehensive picture of the organization's current state of adoption.

Both our research and experience also point to the value of developing an informatics focus to drive improvements in healthcare delivery through technology. This means abandoning the old mental models and traditional boundaries that separate IT from healthcare. Clinical representatives should be actively involved, and they should lead the adoption of clinical systems rather than allowing IT to take the initiative with the project. The IT leadership and team are critical to the success, but only clinicians can truly own the decisions that relate to how care is delivered. In our experience, we know the value of creating an informatics department and ensuring that key representatives serve on steering committees and participate in work groups. Having an informatics focus diminishes resistance, improves workflows, fosters proficiency, and more.

We also learned the value of choosing partners who are willing to invest in your organization. Whether with your IT vendor or another healthcare organization, these strategic relationships can help ease the burdens of adoption and make it easier to achieve. Partners are often a valuable asset when organizations lack the ability or specialization to focus on a key area of adoption.

A lot has changed since we wrote the first edition seven years ago, but one thing hasn't: the value of adopting healthcare IT systems, rather than simply implementing them. Technology doesn't create safer or better care when it is installed, but it has tremendous potential to drive safe, secure, and shared information across the continuum of care when it is thoughtfully used, improved, and optimized. It's an exciting time in our journey, but we have important work to do and it is worth doing. The final words of our first edition remain relevant: *the prescription for lasting adoption isn't a pill, it is a regimen that requires discipline and hard work, but it will result in the lasting adoption of EHR systems.*

124

R E F E R E N C E S

Aldrich, C. (2000). The Justification of IT Training. Gartner Research Note DF-11-3614. Retrieved from http://clarkaldrich.blogspot.com/2007/01/clark-aldrich-bio.html

Amarasingham, R., Plantinga, L., Diener-West, M., Gaskin, D., Powe, N. (2009, January 26). Clinical information technologies and inpatient outcomes: a multiple hospital study. *Archives of Internal Medicine*, 169(2):108-114.

American Medical Informatics Assocation (AMIA). (2006, June 13). A Roadmap for National Action on Clinical Decision Support. Retrieved from http://www.amia.org/inside/initiatives/cds.

American Society for Training and Development (ASTD). (2009). Annual Survey. Retrieved from http://maamodt.asp.radford.edu/HR%20Statistics/dollars_spent_on_training.htm

Asbjörnson, K. (2008, January). Conversation with Charles Fred on Exploring Inspired Leadership Through Music. http://www.inspireimagineinnovate.com/Inspiring-Performance.asp

Bazzoli, Fred. (2016, August 15). The 6 national coordinators who have directed ONC. *Health Data Management*. Retrieved from http://www.healthdatamanagement.com/list/the-6-national-coordinators-who-have-directed-onc

Brown, Alyssa. (2013, November). America's Desire to Shed Pounds Outweighs Effort. *Gallup*. Retrieved from http://www.gallup.com/poll/166082/americans-desire-shed-pounds-outweighs-effort.aspx

Burleson, D. (2001, August 16). Four Factors that Shape the Cost of ERP. Retrieved from http://www.dba-oracle.com/art_erp_factors.htm

Catlin, A., Cowen, C. History of Health Spending in US, 1960-2013. *Centers for Medicare and Medicaid Services*. Retrieved from: https://www.cms.gov/Research-Statistics-Data-and-Systems/Statistics-Trends-and-Reports/NationalHealthExpendData/Downloads/HistoricalNHEPaper.pdf

Centers for Disease Control (CDC), National Center for Health Statistics (NCHS). (2014). Obesity and Overweight. Retrieved from http://www.cdc.gov/nchs/fastats/obesity-overweight.htm

Centers for Medicare and Medicaid Services (CMS). (2014). National Health Expenditure Data. Retrieved from https://www.cms.gov/research-statistics-data-and-systems/statistics-trends-and-reports/nationalhealthexpenddata/nhe-fact-sheet.html

Chatham, Lea. (2015, August 17). EHR Critical for ICD-10 Success. *Getting Paid*. Retrieved from http://gettingpaid.kareo.com/getting-paid/2015/08/ehr-critical-for-icd-10-success/

Chen, C., Garrido, T., Chock, D., Okawa, G., Liang, L. (2009). The Kaiser Permanente Electronic Health Record: Transforming and Streamlining Modalities of Care. *Health Affairs, 28(2)*, 323-333.

Collier, Robert. (2015, January 6). National Physician Survey: EMR Use at 75%. *CMAJ*. 187(1): E17-E18. doi: 10.1503/cmaj.109-4957

Congress of the United States, Congressional Budget Office (CBO). (2008, May). Evidence on the Costs and Benefits of Health Information Technology: A CBO Paper.

CoverMD. (2009). Electronic Medical Records: A Way to Save Money on Your Malpractice Insurance. Retrieved from www.covermd.com/resources/electronic-medical-records-medmal-insurance.aspx

Florida Medical Quality Assurance, Inc. (FMQAI). (2008). Physician Practice Resource Manual: Doctor's Office Quality – Information Technology – 8th Scope of Work, August 1, 2005-July 31, 2008.

Fred, C. (2002). *Breakaway.* Jossey-Bass: San Francisco.

Gladwell, M. (2002). *The Tipping Point: How Little Things Can Make a Big Difference.* Little Brown and Company: New York.

Glicksman, Eve. (2013, May). Wanting it All: A New Generation of Doctors Places Higher Value on Work-Life Balance. *Association of American Medical Colleges.* Retrieved from https://www.aamc.org/ newsroom/reporter/462176/work-life.html

Grieger, D., Cohen, S., Krusch, D. (2007, February 28). A Pilot Study to Document the Return on Investment for Implementing an Ambulatory Electronic Health Record at an Academic Medical Center. *Journal of the American College of Surgeons*, 205(1), 89-96. doi:10.1016/j. jamcollsurg.2007.02.074

Haugen, H. CHIME Focus Group. (2012). *The College of Health Information Management Executives.*

Haugen, H., Tran, Z., Wyatt, H., Barry, M., Hill, J. (2007, December). Using Telehealth to Increase Participation in Weight Maintenance Programs. *Obesity* 15(12), 3067–3077. doi: 10.1038/oby.2007.365

Hessels, A., Flynn, L., Cimiotti, J., Bakken, S., Gershon, R. (2015, November 1). Impact of Health Information Technology on the Quality of Patient Care. *OJNI* 19. Retrieved from http://www.himss.org/ impact-heath-information-technology-quality-patient-care

Himmelstein, D., Jun, M., Busse, R., Chevreul, K., Geissler, A., et al. (2014, September). A Comparison of Hospital Administration Costs in Eight Nations: US Costs Exceed Others by Far. *Health Affairs* 33(9), 1586-1594. doi: 10.1377/hlthaff.2013.1327

James, R. (2009, June 10). Jim Collins: How Mighty Companies Fall. *TIME Magazine.* Retrieved from http://www.time.com/time/business/article/0,8599,1903713,00.html

Jang, Y., Lortie, M., Sanche, S. (2014, September). Return on investment in electronic health records in primary care practices: A mixed-method study. *JMIR Medical Informatics*. 2(2), e25. doi: 10.2196/medinform.3631.

Jha, A., Ferris, T., Donelan, K., DesRoches, C., Shields, A., et al. (2006, October 11). How common are electronic health records in the United States? A summary of the evidence. *Health Affairs*, 25(6), w496-507. doi: 10.1377/hlthaff.25.w496

Kazley, A., Simpson, A., Simpson, K., Teufel, R. (2014, Jun 1). Association of electronic health records with cost savings in a national sample. *American Journal of Managed Care*. 20(6), e183-190. Retrieved from http://www.ajmc.com/journals/issue/2014/2014-vol20-n6/Association-of-Electronic-Health-Records-With-Cost-Savings-in-a-National-Sample/

Kolb, David A. (1984). *Experiential Learning*. Prentice Hall: New Jersey.

Kramer, F., Jeffery, R., Forster, J., Snell, M. (1989). Long-term follow-up of behavioral treatment for obesity: patterns of weight regain among men and women. *International Journal of Obesity and Related Metabolic Disorders*, 13, 123-136.

Massachusetts Technology Cooperative, New England Healthcare Institute (NEHI). (2008). Saving Lives, Saving Money: the imperative for computerized physician order entry in Massachusetts hospitals. Retrieved from http://www.nehi.net/publications/8/saving_lives_saving_money_the_imperative_for_computerized_physician_order_entry_in_massachusetts_hospitals

Makary, M., Daniel, M. (2016, May 3). Medical error – the third leading cause of death in the US. *BMJ*. 3, 353, i2139. Retrieved from http://www.bmj.com/content/353/bmj.i2139 doi: 10.1136/bmj.i2139

Medical Economics. (2016). Top Ten Challenges Facing Physicians in
2016. *Modern Medicine Network*. Retrieved from http://medicaleco-
nomics.modernmedicine.com/medical-economics/news/top-10-chal-
lenges-facing-physicians-2016?page=0,1

Miliard, M. (2015, July 24). Clinical decision support: no longer just a
nice-to-have. *Healthcare IT News*. Retrieved from http://www.healthca-
reitnews.com/news/clinical-decision-support-no-longer-just-nice-have

Nationwide Health Information Network (NHIN). (2009, July 17).
Overview. Retrieved from http://healthit.hhs.gov/portal/server.pt?o
pen=512&objID=1142&parentname=CommunityPage&parentid=2&
mode=2&in_hi_userid=10741&cached=true

Office of the National Coordinator on Health Information Technology.
(2015, December). Hospitals that have Demonstrated Meaningful Use
through Medicare EHR Incentive Program. Retrieved from http://
dashboard.healthit.gov/dashboards/hospitals-medicare-meaningful-
use.php

Office of the National Coordinator on Health Information Technology.
(2015). Non-federal Acute Care Hospital Electronic Health Record
Adoption. Retrieved from http://dashboard.healthit.gov/quickstats/
pages/FIG-Hospital-EHR-Adoption.php

Office of the National Coordinator on Health Information Technology.
(2015). Office-based Physician Electronic Health Record Adoption.
Retrieved from http://dashboard.healthit.gov/quickstats/pages/
physician-ehr-adoption-trends.php

Office of the National Coordinator on Health Information Technology.
(2015). Percent of Hospitals, By Type, that Possess Certified Health
IT. Retrieved from http://dashboard.healthit.gov/quickstats/pages/
certified-electronic-health-record-technology-in-hospitals.php

Senge, P. (1994). *The Fifth Discipline*. Doubleday: New York.

Silow-Carroll, S., Edwards, J., Rodin, D. (2012, July). Using Electronic Health Records to Improve Quality and Efficiency: The Experiences of Leading Hospitals. *The Commonwealth Fund*. Retrieved from http://www.commonwealthfund.org/~/media/files/publications/issue-brief/2012/jul/1608_silowcarroll_using_ehrs_improve_quality.pdf

Sockolow, P., Bowles, K., Adelsberger, M., Chittams, J., Liao, C. (2014, April 30). Impact of homecare electronic health record on timeliness of clinical documentation, reimbursement, and patient outcomes. *Applied Clinical Informatics*. (5)2, 445-462. doi: 10.4338/ACI-2013-12-RA-0106

THINKMAP Visual Thesaurus. (2016). Retrieved from http://www.visual thesaurus.com/

Virapongse, A., Bates, D., Shi, P., Jenter, C., Volk, L., et al. (2008, November 24). Electronic health records and malpractice claims in office practice. *Archives of Internal Medicine*, 168(21), 2362-2367.

Wadden, T. (1993). Treatment of obesity by moderate and severe caloric restriction: Results of clinical research trials. *Annals of Internal Medicine*, 119, 688-693.

Wheatley, M. (2000, June 1). ERP Training Stinks. *CIO Magazine.* Retrieved from http://www.cio.com/article/148900/ERP_Training_Stinks

Wolinsky, Howard. (2016, July 23). With MACRA looming, doctors can't afford waiting to plumb its intricacies. *Modern Healthcare*. Retrieved from http://www.modernhealthcare.com/article/20160723/MAGAZINE/307239981/with-macra-looming-doctors-cant-afford-waiting-to-plumb-its

LITERATURE REVIEW

Adopting an EHR will improve the organization's quality of care, patient safety and efficiency

We have the opportunity to transform healthcare by providing access to comprehensive medical information that is secure, standardized and shared. A significant body of literature confirms the value of electronic health records (EHRs) in improving patient safety, improving coordination of care, enhancing documentation, reducing administrative inefficiencies, facilitating clinical decision-making and adherence to evidence-based clinical guidelines (Chen et al, 2009; Massachusetts Technology Cooperative, 2008; Amarasingham et al, 2009). This literature review provides some strong evidence for improved clinical and financial outcomes.

131

Improved quality of care and patient safety

Improved quality of care and patient safety is often the primary driver for EHR adoption. Clinicians strive to provide the highest quality of care and to be vigilant in ensuring the safety of our patients. Yet a recent study indicates that as many as 251,000 people die each year from medical errors, a staggering statistic to comprehend (Makary and Daniel, 2016). In commercial aviation, this would be the equivalent of nearly three medium-sized airliners crashing every day. Despite our commitment to patient safety, because we are human and because healthcare is extraordinarily complex, taking advantage of improvements in error rates associated with EHR adoption is not something we can afford to pass by.

There is much healthcare can learn from the aviation industry. The Federal Aviation Administration (FAA) mandated Crew Resource Management (CRM) training in 1992. This human factors training focuses on error prevention, recognition and management through teamwork, communication and procedural protocols, and has been a major contributor to a dramatic reduction in commercial aviation accidents.

An EHR can provide analogous benefits to healthcare organizations. It can contribute to patient safety and quality care by preventing errors (drug-drug interactions), recognizing and helping providers manage errors by alerting them to potential complications of treatment (drug allergies) and providing electronic procedural protocols by flagging abnormal laboratory results and reminding providers to schedule preventative health screenings.

"The quality of health care could be improved through the use of Clinical Decision Support (CDS) systems to remind physicians to schedule tests, help diagnose complicated conditions, and more effectively implement appropriate protocols for treatment (Congressional Budget Office, 2008)."

A recent study found that high levels of EHR adoption improve patient outcomes such as decreasing length of stay and hospital readmissions (Hessels, 2016). Evidence suggests that healthcare providers also perceive that EHRs improve patient outcomes. In a recent survey of 10,000 Canadian providers, 65 percent reported that EHR systems improve patient care significantly, and less than 5 percent reported that EHRs have a negative impact on quality of care. Respondents identified the benefits of EHRs as better access to patient information and lab results, alerts for medication errors and reminders for preventative care (Collier, 2015). Through EHR systems, providers are now able to access the right information at the right time to improve the quality and safety of care.

Enhanced documentation

EHR systems enhance the efficiency, completeness, and accuracy of documentation. One study found that EHR use increases the productivity and timeliness of note documentation, as well as billing for reimbursement (Sockolow, 2014). Participants in the study experienced a significant drop in Days to Medicare claims, from 100 to 30. Additionally, the features and functionality of EHR systems are making it easier for providers to comply with new legislation and regulations. The International Statistical Classification of Diseases and Related Health Problems, 10th revision (ICD-10) has significantly increased the need for more complete and accurate clinical documentation (Chatham, 2015). To comply with ICD-10, EHR systems are helping providers by offering templates, coding tools, and electronic superbills that improve charge capture. Accurate charge capture is critical to the financial success of healthcare organizations.

Cost Savings and Improved Operational Efficiency

Today, about 25 percent of US hospital dollars go to healthcare administrative costs (Himmelstein et al, 2014). We have an opportunity to decrease the cost of healthcare dramatically simply by reducing operational inefficiencies.

EHR systems are a powerful tool for cost savings and revenue enhancement. A recent analysis of 550 U.S. hospitals found that advanced EHR systems reduce the cost per patient admission by nearly 10 percent (Kazley et al, 2014). Some evidence also indicates that providers using EHRs are less likely to have paid malpractice claims (Virapongse et al, 2008), and many insurers offer premium credits between 2 and 5 percent for EHR users (CoverMD, 2009). Additionally, enhanced communication and care coordination, fewer duplicative tests, and more efficient interactions with patients are just a few of the operational efficiencies gained through an EHR (Silow-Carroll, 2012).

The combination of cost savings and increased revenue provides a positive return on investment for an EHR. One study examined the EHR implementations of 17 primary care practices, which achieved the breakeven point for recovery of initial and ongoing cumulative costs in 10 months (Jang, 2014). The findings represent an improvement from prior findings, which found the breakeven point occurred in 16 months with subsequent annual savings of $10,000 per provider (Grieger et al, 2007).

Facilitating CDS and Adherence to Evidence-Based Clinical Guidelines

Clinical Decision Support (CDS) systems are becoming increasingly important as providers face advancements in clinical research and new legislative regulations and requirements (Miliard, 2015). Just keeping abreast of the explosion of new research and treatments is a daunting task, not to mention putting them into practice. It is literally impossible for the human brain to assimilate and apply this continually burgeoning amount of new medical information. For example, the number of medical journal articles has increased from 200,000 to 800,000 since 1970. These changes are increasing the importance of using CDS to improve quality of care. A robust CDS module in an EHR encompasses a variety of tools and interventions, such as computerized alerts, reminders, clinical guidelines, order sets, patient reports and dashboards, documentation templates, diagnostic support and clinical workflow tools (American Medical Informatics Association, 2006). CDS is often the last component of an EHR to be adopted because of the complexity, time investment, effort to gain organizational consensus and clinician resistance to "cookbook medicine"; however, most providers do recognize the value of timely, accurate and easy to access clinical knowledge.

135

How the organization chooses to customize and maintain the module will enhance or degrade its functionality. Excessive or inappropriate alerts and reminders can impede adoption. CDS brings tremendous potential value to organizations committed to fine-tuning the application. Like all technology, the content put in dictates the quality of the result.

A healthy dose of skepticism will serve us well as we review the EHR literature, not because it is misleading, but because it doesn't tell the whole story. Despite the promises of an EHR system, why do we continue to hear stories of end-user resistance, applications that experience configuration issues, workflow struggles, higher than expected costs and lower than expected revenues, increases in staffing and worse quality metrics? *The disconnect between the evidence in the literature and our real-world experiences is borne in the assumption that implementing an EHR and adopting an EHR are synonymous.*

The differences between implementing and adopting an EHR are evident when one examines data from the College of Health Information Management Executives (CHIME). These data show

the gap between implementation and adoption across several key functions of clinical information systems. The rate of adoption is significantly lower than the rate of implementation, illustrating that installing an EHR doesn't lead to adopting the application for the clinical benefit of users. The more complex functions, such as Computerized Provider Order Entry (CPOE) and Clinical Decision Support (CDS), have the biggest gap in adoption because they require significant changes in workflow. While 73 percent of healthcare organizations have an EHR installed that is capable of CPOE, only 44 percent of providers have adopted it. Similarly, only 41 percent of providers have adopted CDS despite 84 percent of healthcare organizations having systems installed with CDS (Haugen, CHIME Focus Group, 2012).

Heather A. Haugen, Ph.D
Charles L. Fred

The authors remain relentlessly passionate about the adoption of healthcare technology. Their extensive experience in helping organizations improve outcomes through technology has led them to discover the best practices for optimizing clinical information systems. The authors have witnessed the outcomes of poor adoption and remain committed to helping organizations successfully surmount this challenge, ultimately making healthcare safer and more efficient.

Dr. Heather Haugen is the CEO and Managing Director of The Breakaway Group, A Xerox Company, where she has served in an executive leadership role for over 15 years. Dr. Haugen brings a research focus to the adoption of health information technology. She has more than 20 years of research experience in both the academic and private sectors. Dr. Haugen regularly speaks at national conferences and publishes in academic and industry publications. She has published in numerous health and medical journals, including the *Journal of the American Dietetic Association, Journal of the American College of Nutrition, ADVANCE for Health Information Executives* and *Healthcare Informatics*. Dr. Haugen also blogs on behalf of Xerox's Healthcare Provider Solutions division on areas focused on overcoming the challenges of HIT adoption across the industry. In addition to *Beyond Implementation: A Prescription for Lasting EMR Adoption* (2010), Dr. Haugen is the author of *Beyond Coding: How ICD-10 Will Transform Clinical Documentation* (2012). As a result of the research published in Beyond Implementation, she was selected as a 2010 Finalist for Champions in Healthcare.

Dr. Haugen holds a faculty position at the University of Colorado Denver – Anschutz Medical Center as the Track Director of Health Information Technology, where she actively mentors doctoral students and teaches courses.

Dr. Haugen earned her doctorate in health information technology from the University of Colorado Anschutz Medical Campus. She earned her Master of Science degree in clinical nutrition from Colorado State University, and her Bachelor's degree in biological sciences from the University of Denver.

◆

Charles Fred is a best-selling author, and a serial entrepreneur. He has devoted over three decades of his life discovering new ways for professionals to acquire skills necessary to compete in today's knowledge-thirsty economy. Considered a pioneer in the e-learning industry, Charles has founded and led a number of successful companies that provide learning technologies and services. His best-selling book, *Breakaway,* is credited with transforming learning strategies within service organizations across the globe.

In 2000, Charles founded The Breakaway Group, one of the nation's fastest growing companies, to transform how healthcare providers learn and adopt new technologies. Xerox acquired The Breakaway Group in 2011 and in the process Charles became President of their healthcare group, providing technology and services worldwide.

Today, as the CEO of Modern Teacher, Charles is taking his healthcare expertise and experience and devoting his time to help teachers reinvent the classroom. Charles is also the founder of The Reignite Group, a research-based firm dedicated to helping entrepreneurs make the transition to chief executives and discover important know-how to build lasting enterprises.

Charles is a long-time resident of Colorado and avid outdoor enthusiast. He and his wife, Julie, dedicate much of their time with their family, mentoring young people and entrepreneurs, and giving back to the community.

The **Breakaway** Group
A Xerox Company

For over 16 years, The Breakaway Group, A Xerox Company has been revolutionizing how healthcare learns, implements, and adopts new health information technology. With experience helping over 1 million professionals optimize the use of health IT systems, we guarantee that our customized, scalable, repeatable learning solution will establish user proficiency in any health IT application. The Breakaway Method™ supports healthcare organizations in adoption of new workflow applications 60% to 80% faster than traditional classroom education.

By helping end users adopt new software applications quickly and easily, our solution helps providers have more time for patient care, healthcare executives see improved financial outcomes, and those leading technology implementations experience less stress.

To learn more about The Breakaway Group please visit
www.thebreakawaygroup.com
or contact us at
303-483-4300.

140

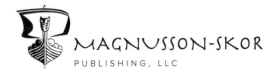

MAGNUSSON-SKOR
PUBLISHING, LLC

Magnusson-Skor Publishing.
Helping Discover and Unleash Your Point of View.

At Magnusson-Skor Publishing, we believe in the power of a point of view. Our goal is to help our clients gain credibility, thought leadership, and recognition in their industry by crafting or unraveling their point of view for dramatic impact on their success. Since 2001, our dedicated team has brought the talent, time, and capacity that has enabled our clients to craft their point of view into best-selling books, conferences, keynote speeches, and more.

To learn more about Magnusson-Skor Publishing, visit:
www.magnussonskor.com

141

PRINTED IN THE UNITED STATES

9 780984 205141